Heart

of the

MATTER

A Journey to Faith

ENDORSEMENTS

In this moving memoir, the author masterfully weaves together both her health and faith journeys, inviting readers to walk alongside her as she comes to find the comfort and peace that a relationship with God provides in the midst of a challenging disease diagnosis. The narrative is both raw and uplifting, as the author navigates her struggles with grace and humor, transforming moments of hardship into powerful stories intertwined with lessons on faith. With vivid storytelling and emotional depth, this book is a testament to the strength that a life deeply rooted in Christ can provide and the beauty of embracing one's own journey.

—Erin Pope, Operations Director, The Grove Church.

Ms. Edge has written a deeply personal book about her health journey and how she came to Christ because of it. Anyone who has suffered a devastating illness—or who has loved someone with one—will find comfort in her story of triumphing over the odds. As a bonus, the book contains profiles of a half-dozen people in the Bible who overcame adversity and fulfilled God's will for their lives.

—Sandra Bretting, author of *Unfit to Serve*, *Shameless Persistence*, *The Safecracker's Secret*, and six cozy mysteries.

Laura Edge does a masterful job in telling her heart transplant journey in her book *Heart of the Matter*! She beautifully walks you through the physical and emotional ups and downs of heart disease in a way that is very compelling and informative all the while telling you her personal story that is moving and genuine!

—Tracie Woodward, women's ministry director.

Heart of the Matter is a compelling memoir that beautifully weaves the moving stories of a medical journey and a faith journey together. Laura's honest vulnerability shines through as she chronicles her battle with heart disease and her life-changing experience of receiving a heart transplant. Her ability to connect the raw emotion of her crisis with her devotion to God—who holds her life in his hands—challenges readers to think about how they can trust God in deeper ways themselves. This book is a testament to the faithfulness of both a caring God and caring people. *Heart of the Matter* reminds readers of how valuable life is, while also offering hope for anyone facing a serious crisis. Laura's journey will touch your soul and leave you with a renewed sense of gratitude and wonder!

—Whitney Hopler, author of *Wake Up to Wonder* and *Wonder Through the Year: A Daily Devotional for Every Year*.

Heart

of the

MATTER

A Journey to Faith

Laura B. Edge

COPYRIGHT NOTICE

Library Cataloging Data

Names: Edge, Laura B. (Laura B. Edge)

Heart of the Matter: A Journey to Faith / Laura B. Edge

202 p. 23cm × 15cm (9in × 6in.)

ISBN-13: 9798891343528 (paperback) | 9798891343535 (trade paperback) | 9798891343542 (e-book)

Key Words: Women Christian living memoir heart transplant; Inspirational wife mom surviving heart disease; Self-reflection women's issues Christian faith; Jesus prayer true story heart transplant wife mom; Motherhood marriage Christian health crisis growth; Biblical wisdom prayer journey health recovery; Spirituality Bible memoir Christian woman survivalLibrary of Congress Control Number: 2025933620 Nonfiction

DEDICATION

To the family who donated the heart of their loved one, my new heart. Thank you will never be enough.

TABLE OF CONTENTS

ACKNOWLEDGMENTS

I am profoundly grateful to the many, many people who walked beside me or carried me on my journey to heart health. To my husband Gerry, the love of my life and my best friend, thank you for your unwavering support and for the countless hours you spent by my side at the hospital. Thank you for giving me strength when I had none. Thank you for all the times you said, "How can I help?"

My heartfelt thanks to my beautiful sons, Jeremy and Jonathan. I understand miracles are possible because of you. Thank you for giving me a lifetime of joy. Your love gives me hope and a reason to fight for life. Thank you, Dana, for your sweet encouragement to me and the entire Edge clan. You held us together with your unique blend of kindness and strength. Thank you, Darren, for the hours you sat with your dad in the hospital waiting room giving him support when he needed it most. Thank you, Colleen, for your calm thoughtfulness and expert clarification of medical jargon. I love you all.

To my sister Kathy, thank you for listening and for your willingness to do whatever it takes to help, regardless of the situation. You are my safe port in turbulent waters. To

Chris, your bravery and tenacity are an inspiration, and your wit and sense of humor never fail to lighten a room. Thank you for showing me how to put one foot in front of the other when I'd rather just sleep.

Thank you will never be enough for my brilliant team of doctors. First and foremost, Dr. Strickman, an exceptional cardiologist and a magnificent human being. Thank you for enabling me to thrive through many long years of heart disease. You are the best! Thank you to my heart transplant surgical and postsurgical team, who tirelessly worked with kindness, empathy, and excellence to save my life—Dr. Shafii, Dr. Mattar, Dr. Nair, and Dr. Taimeh. To Elane Biles, my transplant coordinator and the cardiac nursing staff, thank you for caring for grumpy patients with compassion and excellence.

I have been blessed to have dear friends walk beside me through the years—Diane Oxner, Frances Hadjigeorge, Rosemary Saye, and Linda Lynch. Your friendship has sustained me, and I call myself fortunate to have each of you in my life. To all the people who took the time to send an encouraging note or card, I saved each one, and they absolutely brightened my darkest days. Thank you to my neighborhood friends, church friends, teaching friends, line dance friends, tap dance friends, and women's prison ministry friends. Thank you, Karen Fahel, for your unfailing encouragement and willingness to help in any way, large and small. I want to thank Gregg and Lisa Van Kampen, my church family, and all the people who prayed for me during my heart transplant journey.

I am grateful to my fellow writers, Miriam King and Chris Mandelski, patient readers of early drafts, for their valuable suggestions, and to my entire critique group, Doris Fisher, Monica Vavra, Tammy Waldrop, and Lynne

Kelly. Your support and enthusiasm helped me find my voice and encouraged me to keep writing. I want to thank Marvin Keown for the many times he brought God's Word to life for me and for making sure my words stayed faithful to biblical truth. A huge thank you goes out to my editor, Susan Hobbs, for finding mistakes I didn't see and to my publisher, Elk Lake Publishing, for taking a chance on my story.

I also want to thank every person who has donated their loved one's organs. Amid profound sadness, you found the strength to donate lifesaving organs to complete strangers. To all of you, thank you from every piece of my old and new heart.

And finally, thank you to Jesus Christ, my Lord and Savior, for holding my heart in your hands and allowing it to keep beating.

PART I

CHAPTER ONE:
CARDIO WHAT?

In this world you will have trouble. But take heart! I have overcome the world. (John 16:33)

My heart broke for the first time when I was thirty-nine years old. I didn't see it coming, and with the suddenness of a bomb, my life exploded into fragments it took years to reassemble.

It started on our first family vacation. My husband Gerry and I planned to fly our six-year-old son Jeremy and his five-year-old brother Jonathan to Florida to frolic in the sun at the Happiest Place on Earth. The boys were counting down the days until we hopped on an airplane and flew from Houston, Texas, to Disney World in Orlando, Florida.

The trip started out rocky. A few days before we were scheduled to leave, Jeremy developed an ear infection.

"He'll feel much better after a couple of days of antibiotics," said his pediatrician.

"We're going to Disney World next week," I said. "Will he be okay to fly?"

The doctor shook his head. "No, he shouldn't fly until the infection has cleared completely. The change in altitude on an airplane could rupture his eardrum."

"But our tickets are nonrefundable."

"You can still take your vacation," the doctor said. "You just can't fly."

It was too late to cancel the trip, so we moved to Plan B: driving from Houston to Orlando. The trip would take a couple of days, but by then the antibiotics would kick in and Jeremy would feel better. To soften the boys' disappointment at not being able to fly in an airplane for the first time, we described the drive as an adventure. "Imagine all the cool stuff we'll get to see on the way! It'll be so much fun! Whoo-hoo!"

In 1993, we didn't have cell phones, so we couldn't use GPS or online navigation apps. But we belonged to AAA, an emergency car service. They planned trip routes and provided maps to their customers as part of their service. We called AAA, gave them our itinerary, and a day later, a package of maps arrived in the mail with highlighted instructions showing each road to take to get us from Houston to Orlando. The original GPS.

We had no handheld video games, DVD players, or MP3 players, so I picked up lots of coloring books and shiny new boxes of crayons. We arranged a cozy nest in the back seat of our car and loaded it with all kinds of snacks, a ton of children's books, books on tape, and our stash of coloring books. The boys settled into the back seat, Jeremy at one window, Jonathan at the other, with the goodies between them, and off we went on our first family vacation.

The boys were amazing in the car. They had never been on a long road trip and were happy as could be coloring in their new coloring books for hours at a time. When that grew old, I read to them while Gerry drove. We listened to *Hank the Cowdog* on tape, played "I Spy with My Little Eyes," took naps, and searched the roadside for cool scenery. The hours flew, and before anyone got car cranky, we were checking into our hotel at Disney World. Jeremy's doctor was right. By the time we got to Orlando, his earache was gone, and he felt great.

We had a blast running from one ride to the next, eating junk food, hugging Disney characters, snapping pictures, and laughing until our jaws ached. In those days, the characters strolled around the park, and children could walk up to them, or in the case of Jeremy and Jonathan, run, get their signatures, and chat with them for as long as they liked. Getting signatures from all the Disney characters became a quest, and Jeremy and Jonny carried their autograph books like priceless treasures. We all fell under Disney's magic spell, and in spite of the rocky start, our first family vacation was a rousing success.

Except for one thing. Somewhere along the way, I picked up a cough.

"I must have caught Jeremy's bug," I told Gerry. "I'll check it out when we get home."

Back in Houston, I went to see our general practitioner. She told me I had an upper respiratory infection and wrote a prescription for an antibiotic. I took the antibiotic, and each day I felt worse instead of better. Sleep was impossible because when I lay down, I coughed so much it felt like I was drowning. Even though I propped myself up with pillows, the deep, hacking cough didn't stop.

As I was not able to sleep in a bed, I spent my nights in a chair in the living room so at least Gerry could get some rest. I didn't have much of an appetite and food tasted like cardboard, so I didn't eat much. But I gained weight. A lot of weight. My body felt fat and puffy, my feet and legs swelled, and wearing underpants hurt my bloated belly. I returned to the doctor to get a stronger prescription.

She ordered a chest x-ray, and it revealed fluid in my lungs. "Pneumonia," she said. "Let's put you in the hospital for a couple of days, pump some antibiotics into you, and knock this thing out."

No, no, no, no, no! I thought. *No hospital. I've been in more than enough hospitals to last a lifetime. I DO NOT like hospitals.*

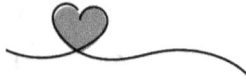

My aversion to hospitals began thirteen years earlier when I spent countless hours visiting my sister, Chris, in one hospital after another. The youngest of five children in our boisterous Italian Irish family, Chris had been the most adorable baby I'd ever seen—curly blonde hair, sparkly blue eyes, and a tiny dimple in her left cheek. I was ten years old when she was born, and I cherished her as my own living doll. With four other children to care for, Mom was more than willing to let me take over baby chores, and Chris and I formed a lifelong unbreakable bond.

Chris was a senior in high school when she got sick. Everything she ate came right back out, and she lost a ton of weight. Doctors ran tests, floated theories, and tried different types of medicines, but they couldn't figure out what was wrong with her. Nothing they tried had any effect.

Chris spent weeks in the hospital as various doctors tried to diagnose her illness. She was my parents' youngest child, and her illness nearly broke my softhearted father. A charismatic salesman who owned his own company, Frank's typical confident ease evaporated the second he walked into a hospital. Watching one of his children suffer was almost more than he could bear. So, Mom took control. She yanked Chris out of the local hospital and transferred her to Houston's downtown medical center under the care of Dr. Red Duke, one of the city's premier surgeons.

Dr. Duke ran Hermann Hospital and developed their famous Trauma Center and Life Flight programs. He was a Houston icon and became a hero to our family. Tall and lanky, with a bushy mustache and a Texas drawl, Dr. Duke was totally Texan. He called Chris "puddin' head" and possessed the rare combination of a down-to-earth demeanor and a brilliant mind. Dr. Duke discovered Chris had Crohn's disease, an incurable condition that destroys the digestive system. He performed an intestinal resection, where he removed the diseased portions of her small and large intestines and sewed the healthy pieces back together.

Chris spent the remainder of her senior year in the hospital, slowly recovered, graduated from high school, and attended college the following fall. But her Crohn's disease reared its ugly head every few years and wreaked havoc on her life. She lived in an apartment near me in Houston, and when the disease returned again and again, I'd call an ambulance to take her to the hospital and cringe in the hallway as I listened to her scream in pain. She had countless surgeries, each one cutting away portions of her large and small intestine, and I learned to fear hospitals as places of torture and pain.

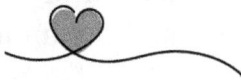

Now, as I sat in my doctor's office and listened to her try to convince me to check myself into a hospital, every horrid hospital memory from my sister's illness slammed into my head and left me reeling.

I took a deep breath, looked at the doctor, and tried to steady my voice. "I can't go into a hospital," I said. "I have two little boys who need me at home. Can't you give me a stronger prescription?"

"You're already on one of the strongest antibiotics available," the doctor said. "The only thing stronger is given through an IV. You'll only be in the hospital for a couple of days. This is the quickest and easiest way to make you feel better."

Easier for you, maybe, but absolutely not easier for me.

I tried to convince Gerry the hospital was a bad idea, but he agreed with the doctor. "Two days, honey," he said. "I've got the boys covered. Give it two days."

Famous last words.

I grumbled my way to the local hospital, and the cough grew worse. Doctors pumped bags and bags of antibiotics into my veins. They added breathing treatments and asked me to suck into a plastic cylinder ten times an hour to strengthen my lungs. I hated that canister with a maniacal loathing. It hurt my chest and made the cough worse. Days passed, then a week. I gained more weight, grew short of breath, and felt like hammered mud.

My doctor called in a bunch of lung specialists to figure out why I wasn't getting better. As the group of physicians hovered around my bed, my hospital frustration boiled over. "Maybe we should try something else," I said. "This doesn't seem to be working."

The doctors shuffled out of my room and huddled in the hallway to whisper and toss around ideas. Then they ordered lots of different types of tests.

An echocardiogram uncovered an alarming discovery: my heart showed some sort of abnormality and was pumping weakly. My doctor urged me to find a cardiologist and transfer to a hospital that specialized in heart disease.

Heart disease? What are you talking about? I don't have heart disease.

But she insisted I needed a cardiologist, and not one of the regular cardiologists at my local hospital. "You need a cardiologist at the medical center who specializes in a disease called cardiomyopathy."

Gerry and I didn't know one cardiologist from another, and we were clueless about where to go in the massive Houston Medical Center complex. We called everyone we knew for help. Friends in the area suggested doctors. My older sister Kathy, a high-ranking executive in New York, used her contacts around the country to research the best cardiologists in Houston and sent us their names. With no internet or Google, we were not able to check out doctors like we do today. By dumb luck, we picked Dr. Neil Strickman at St. Luke's Hospital.

My doctor contacted Dr. Strickman and filled him in on my test results. Gerry and I prepared for my transfer to the downtown hospital and tried to decode the strange-sounding diagnosis.

"What did she call it? Cardiomyopathy?" I asked. "I've never heard of it."

Gerry shook his head. "Me neither."

A bubbly young nurse hung a new bag of medicine on my IV pole and said, "Oh, you know that movie *Beaches* with Bette Midler and Barbara Hershey? That's what Barbara Hershey's character died of."

The room tilted a bit and Gerry and I fell silent.

Did she say, "died of?"

CHAPTER TWO:
MEN & BOYS

"For I know the plans I have for you," declares the Lord, *"plans to prosper you and not to harm you, plans to give you hope and a future." (Jeremiah 29:11)*

I thought about the nurse's remark as I watched her prepare IVs and paperwork for my transfer to St. Luke's Hospital. *This may not be a simple bug after all*, I thought with a feeling of dread. She held out a stack of papers for me to sign.

"These will go with you in the ambulance," she said. "They contain all your test results and blood work."

I nodded and signed. "I'd rather go in my car." I thought the ambulance was unnecessary, embarrassing, and over-the-top dramatic. I couldn't lie down because I coughed nonstop and would have to ride propped up in a sitting position. I could do that in my car.

I glanced at Gerry for support and he nodded. "Yes," he said. "I'd like to take her."

The nurse shook her head. "No, you need to be transported by ambulance. Hospital policy. It should be here in a few minutes."

Gerry stood beside my bed and held my hand. "Then I'd like to ride in the ambulance with her," he said.

"No, that's not allowed. You'll have to follow in your car."

I squeezed Gerry's hand and felt my control slipping away, one hospital rule at a time.

Two young men in crisp blue uniforms maneuvered a tall rolling bed into my room. They strapped me in, attached the IV pole, and wheeled me into a waiting ambulance. One of the paramedics sat beside me as the ambulance zigzagged through traffic. I stared out the back window and looked for Gerry's truck, thankful for the darkness that made me anonymous, and thought about the people I loved. I had no idea what was going through my husband's mind at that moment, but my thoughts instantly jumped to our children and the life Gerry and I had built together. I blocked out the voices of the paramedics, the radio static, the traffic noise, and the deafening roar of worry, confusion, and rising panic inside my head and reflected on all we had shared as a family.

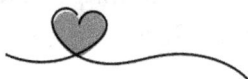

Gerry and I met at an engineering company where he worked as a civil/structural engineer and I worked as a project scheduler. It was my first corporate job after years of teaching middle school math and language arts, and I felt like a wide-eyed rookie. I had to pretend I belonged in my beautiful office in an even more beautiful high-rise building. I wasn't an engineer, didn't know the lingo, and knew I'd have to work hard and learn fast if I was going to survive my first nonteaching job.

Not long after I started with the company, a coworker named Monte invited me to a meeting about a new project. I showed up in my one and only suit, notebook in hand, eager to learn how to do the job they were paying me to do. "Have a seat," said Monte.

As I waited for the engineer to arrive, I thought about the responsibilities that came with my new position. I was learning how to create timelines and schedules for engineers to use as guides to help them complete projects on time and under budget. I was expected to identify the "critical path," the sequence of dependent tasks that determines the most efficient schedule possible to complete a project. I hoped Monte's project wouldn't be too complicated for me to decipher the critical path.

A few minutes later, the engineer arrived, and Monte introduced him as Gerry. We had not seen each other around the office, but that was not surprising in a large corporation with several floors of employees. As I waited for the meeting to begin, Monte grinned and informed us the meeting was a sham. He had noticed Gerry and me around the office and thought we should meet. According to him, we looked like "Barbie and Ken."

Gerry was too cute for his own good—broad shoulders, three-piece suit, meticulously trimmed beard, longish hair, and a killer smile. Definitely dangerous, especially when he turned on the charm. Which he did in Monte's office.

Leaning over the desk, Gerry asked, "What's your phone number?"

I tried to act like a professional and gave him my four-digit work extension. Then I headed to the door.

Gerry wrote down my work extension and smiled. "What about your home number?"

My cheeks flamed with embarrassment. *What is wrong with you? I'm trying to be a serious businesswoman here. Give me a break!*

With as much dignity as I could muster, I glared at him and said, "I'm not giving you my phone number. I don't even know you." Then I walked out of Monte's office.

Gerry claims that was the moment he knew we would marry and spend our lives together.

It took me a while to agree with him, but he was right. We were married two years later.

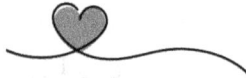

As the ambulance sped through traffic a horn blasted on the freeway and pulled me out of my memories. I stared out the back window and searched for Gerry's truck in the flow of cars behind us. He had sacrificed so much to give me the life we shared. I knew he must be frantic with worry. I thought about our beautiful children, Jeremy and Jonathan, and Gerry's children from his first marriage, Dana and Darren. They lived in Tucson, Arizona, with their mother and her new husband, but they were very much in Texas in our hearts.

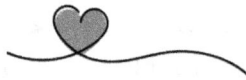

After his first marriage ended, the pain of leaving Dana and Darren was so intense, Gerry had a vasectomy to ensure he'd never father another child. When we married, I didn't think it was a big deal. My life was happy with Gerry, and I didn't need children to make our marriage complete.

But when I reached my thirties, my biological clock started ticking, and I knew my window for bearing a child was rapidly closing. Maybe it was getting to know Dana and Darren or maybe it was the fact that after three years, our marriage had solidified and our love had deepened, but I realized I did want children. I wanted our children.

So, Gerry had a vasectomy reversal, a painful operation to put it mildly. The procedure didn't work. He had another surgery. Then another. Nothing worked, so we started looking into the process of adoption.

Diane, one of my teaching buddies and best friends, had moved from Houston to Memphis, Tennessee, with her husband Brent and their children a few years earlier. Diane and Brent shared a deep, unshakable faith in God, a faith that permeated every aspect of their lives. Diane and Brent knew about our struggle to have a baby and were praying for us. Around this time, Brent made a rare stop home in the middle of the day to pick up something for work. He flipped on the television and saw a doctor on a talk show who claimed to have a 90 percent success rate with vasectomy reversal surgery. Brent told Diane about the doctor, and Diane badgered the television station until they gave her the name and contact information for this wonder doctor.

Gerry and I were skeptical to say the least.

"He claims a 90 percent success rate?" I asked Diane. "How is that possible?"

"I don't know," said Diane. "But it's worth checking out."

Gerry had already suffered through three unsuccessful surgeries. Could I ask him to endure a fourth? What could this St. Louis doctor do that the others hadn't tried? On the other hand, it's hard to ignore 90 percent success. Another compelling reason to check it out was the information came from Diane. She was the most spiritual person I'd ever met and seemed to have a hotline to God. We called the St. Louis doctor, and his office verified Diane's claims. His nurse also told us Dr. Sherman Silber had a three-year waiting list. They put Gerry's name on the list and we settled in for a long wait. I tried to put it out of my mind and hoped my eggs wouldn't dry up before we could get to St. Louis.

A week later, Dr. Silber's office called and said they had a cancellation. Would we like to come to St. Louis the following week for surgery?

We cleaned out our savings account and hopped on an airplane. Gerry had surgery, and I became pregnant with Jeremy three months later.

My mother's name for me, "Sweet Little Laura," died the moment I held Jeremy for the first time. An overwhelming wave of protectiveness invaded every cell of my body. I became a warrior woman, a Navy SEAL, and a charging lioness protecting her cub. I am a nonviolent pacifist by nature, but I knew in that moment I would do anything to protect this precious miracle child. *Anything.* I felt an overwhelming surge of love for my tiny, flawless son.

Gerry and I thought I couldn't get pregnant while I was nursing Jeremy, but we found out that was not true. I became pregnant with Jonathan six months after Jeremy's birth. In a hurry to catch up with his brother, Jonathan made a dramatic entrance into our lives. My labor with Jeremy had been short—three hours from start to finish. When my labor started with Jonathan, it was fast and furious. I knew he would be here soon, but our hospital was an hour away in downtown Houston.

Gerry sped through traffic and hoped to attract a police escort to get us to the hospital in time and spare him the prospect of delivering Jonathan on the side of the freeway. Police officers stopped me all the time for speeding and I had the tickets to prove it, but the day Jonny was born, there wasn't an officer in sight.

When we arrived at the hospital, the staff did not share our concerns about Jonathan's imminent arrival.

"Don't worry, Mrs. Edge," the nurse said. "We have plenty of time. Relax."

Then she checked things out.

"Get a doctor in here!" she screamed into the hallway. "Now!"

A doctor I'd never met took over for the nurse, and Jonathan made his appearance a minute later. The doctor handed Jonny to Gerry, and it was all he could do to hold on to his son. A wiggly ball of energy, Jonathan nearly ended up on the hospital floor. We left the hospital the next morning, thrilled, thankful, and overjoyed with our lively little boy. I felt like the luckiest person in the history of the world.

With two little boys, life was chaotic, and I was having a blast. My parents lived on the other side of Houston, and we enjoyed spending time with them and watching our boys get to know Grandma and Grandpa. A week before Jonathan's first birthday, the phone rang one bright spring morning and time stopped. My dad woke up that morning, walked to the kitchen, poured a glass of milk, sat at the kitchen table, had a massive heart attack, and died. When my mom waltzed into the kitchen several hours later to answer a ringing telephone, she wondered why he wasn't answering the phone. She thought he was asleep.

"Frank, wake up, the phone's ringing," she said.

She tried to wake him, but it was too late. He was gone.

Frank's death affected my mom and each of his five children differently. Mom was in shock and utterly devastated. Shortly after the funeral, she sold the dream house in Houston she and Frank had designed and built together and moved to California where they had spent the early years of their marriage. As she moved so far away so quickly, it felt like we lost both parents at the same time.

The suddenness of my father's death seemed hardest to bear. I thought back to the last time I'd seen him and tried to remember if I'd told him how much I loved him. Did I rush out the door without giving him a hug? Was I preoccupied with Jeremy and Jonathan? His death was too quick. How could a person seem perfectly fine one minute and then drop dead the next? At sixty, Frank was much too young to die, but as my father loathed hospitals, a lingering illness would have been brutal for him. I drew comfort from the realization that dying suddenly at home was the best possible way for his life to end.

Jeremy was two and Jon turned one a few days after the funeral. I grieved my sons would never know the wonderful man who showed me what love looks like. When I came home after the funeral, the television was turned on. I stood in the middle of the living room, stared at the TV, and waited for the news anchor to report my father's death. To me it was the most important event in the world. A gaping hole had opened in the universe and could never be filled. To everyone else on the planet, it was simply a day in May.

That same sense of incredulity washed over me four years later as my ambulance pulled up to St. Luke's Hospital. Heart disease had caused my father's sudden death, and now paramedics were wheeling me into a massive hospital that specialized in the very thing that killed Frank.

CHAPTER THREE:
A WHOLE NEW WORLD

*Be strong and courageous. Do not be afraid; do not be discouraged, for the L*ORD *your God will be with you wherever you go. (Joshua 1:9)*

Gerry later told me the forty-five-minute drive to the medical center was the most scared he'd ever been in his life. The flashing lights and whining siren ignited his fear I'd be dead by the time he got to the hospital.

When we arrived at St. Luke's, a team of cardiologists jumped into action. We met Dr. Strickman, who did not fit my mental image of an eminent cardiologist. With his receding hairline and bushy mustache, he looked like Richard Dreyfuss in hospital scrubs. His team of cardiologists went over my medical history, which wasn't much. I'd been healthy my whole life. Dr. Strickman reviewed the echocardiogram from my local hospital and ordered another, along with what seemed like a billion blood tests.

The results came in the next morning, and Dr. Strickman moved me to a room in cardiac intensive care. The tests confirmed the diagnosis of cardiomyopathy and congestive heart failure. I learned a bunch of fancy heart disease words that described my heart as enlarged and pumping weakly. As a result, my other organs were not getting enough blood flow and my kidneys were failing.

"But I never get sick," I said. "How did I get it?"

Dr. Strickman frowned. "We're not sure. You may have been born with it. A virus may have damaged your heart. We can't pinpoint the exact cause, but the result is a weakened heart muscle."

As I struggled to make sense of his words, a million questions filled my mind. *Is this some kind of mistake? How can a person zip around Disney World hugging Mickey and Minnie one day and find out they have a damaged heart the next? What will this mean for Gerry? For Jeremy and Jonathan? Will I be able to care for them? Will they get it?*

I took a step back from the edge of Panic Cliff and forced myself to focus on what Dr. Strickman was trying to tell me.

"Can I take medicine to fix it?" I asked.

"Yes, we'll certainly try that," he said.

Gerry and I stared at him, mute. *Try that?*

Dr. Strickman left to check on his other patients, and a few of the doctors on his team stayed to answer any questions we might have. After sputtering out a few random queries, we finally got the picture. One of the tests measured my heart's ejection fraction, how much blood the left ventricle pumps out with each heartbeat. A normal heart's ejection fraction is between 55 and 70 percent. Mine was 11. My heart was in bad shape, really bad shape, and the likelihood of a heart as damaged as mine repairing itself was slim. There was a distinct possibility I would not live through the weekend.

I heard the doctors' words, but deep down, I did not believe them. Yes, I felt crummy, so I knew something was wrong. But my heart couldn't be as damaged as the doctors claimed. They must have mixed up my records with another patient. Do these people know what they're doing? Can they be right? *I don't feel like I'm on the brink of death!*

A parade of doctors stopped by my room throughout the day. They ordered a variety of tests and reviewed my medical history in detail to look for clues to my current debilitating condition. They latched on to the fact my father had died of a massive heart attack and tried to determine whether my heart problem was related in some way to his. The hospital staff seemed surprised when they met me. I didn't have high blood pressure or high cholesterol. I wasn't diabetic. I wasn't overweight. I didn't smoke and only drank wine occasionally. I was physically active, and I was in my thirties. I did not fit the mold of a cardiac intensive care patient.

"Have you ever smoked?" asked one of the doctors.

"In high school, but that was a million years ago and didn't last long." I didn't think it was relevant to mention how I got caught smoking my first cigarette in the bathroom of my high school freshman year and was suspended from school for three days. Nor did I share my mom's reaction, "I don't mind you smoking, but why in the world did you do it at school?" Of course, Mom had started chain smoking at fourteen, so she was hardly the person to warn me of the health dangers of cigarettes.

So, smoking was ruled out as the cause of my current medical predicament as were obesity, alcoholism, and drug abuse. The pack of doctors left scratching their heads and went to interrogate other patients.

Someone was always popping into my room in intensive care with medicine, another IV, a new test, or more questions. One of the chattier nurses stayed and sat with me for a while. "I've never seen this before," she said. "There's another woman in her thirties with cardiomyopathy right down the hall."

"How is she doing?" I asked.

The nurse sighed. "Not well."

When the activity in intensive care slowed down, I began to grasp the seriousness of my situation. My mind jumped from the doctors' earnest faces to our children and what my health crisis would mean for them. As I worried about my family and attempted to rein in my scattered thoughts, Gerry reminded me St. Luke's Hospital was the best heart hospital in Houston. "The doctors here know a lot more about heart disease than we do," he said. "We need to calm down, trust them, and do what they say."

"You're right," I said. "Patients surprise doctors all the time and get better when things look grim. I'll follow their treatment plan, beat the odds, and get better."

Gerry nodded. "These are the top guys. They'll figure it out."

I couldn't tell if Gerry was trying to convince me or himself, but my fear receded to a manageable level. My mind began to function again, and I came up with a plan—a plan that had worked for me in the past.

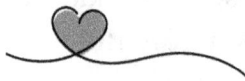

As a child, I attended Immaculate Conception Catholic School in Waukegan, Illinois, a suburb north of Chicago, from first through eighth grades. Instead of science classes, we had religion classes. Several times a week, one of the priests came into our classroom and told us stories about a really cool guy named Jesus. My friend Nikki and I wore frilly white dresses and flowers in our hair for our first Holy

Communion. I didn't have a profound spiritual awakening, but Nikki and I had fun twirling around in our fancy dresses and posing for pictures.

My teachers were nuns, and they made a huge impression on me, especially when they pulled rulers out from under their scary black habits and whacked children on the knuckles for bad behavior. It was confusing. If they were "Brides of Christ," women who were supposed to be holy, kind, and close to God, I did not see examples of God's love in their ruler-wielding behavior.

I walked to school with my friend Mary. We lived on a dead-end street that led into Powell Park. On the other side of the park and down Grand Avenue sat our school. One morning, Mary and I were moseying through the park, in no hurry to get to school. I was ahead of her, at the top of a small hill. She was chatting with a man at the bottom of the hill who reached out, grabbed her arm, and held something against her side. I shifted from one foot to the other. If she didn't move it, we'd be late for school.

Out of nowhere, a small dog flew past me down the hill and circled the pair, barking, growling, and nipping at the man's legs. When he looked down and tried to shoo the dog away, Mary yanked her arm free, raced up the hill, grabbed my hand, and yelled, "Run!"

I fell into step beside her. The look on her face told me not to ask questions, just run. I glanced back and saw the man running too. Racing to catch us. Blind instinct told me this man was up to no good. I had no idea what he wanted, but I knew I needed to get away from him.

We flew across the park, up the concrete steps to Grand Avenue, and down the street to school. We could hear the man's footsteps pounding on the sidewalk behind us, but fear gave us super speed. We burst into school and collapsed in the office. Panting and holding our sides, we told the principal about the man. A group of nuns went outside to see if they could find him, and the principal called the police.

Mary and I became part of an ongoing police investigation. A man matching our park prowler's description had been attempting to abduct young girls in our area. The police were anxious to apprehend the man before he frightened or harmed any other children. To help police identify the man, we went to the police station and looked through books of mug shots. We went to a police lineup where we stood in a small room with a glass window that allowed us to see a row of men but remain unseen to them. We couldn't find the man in the photos or the lineup, and as far as I know, the police never caught him. Mary and I looked for the dog that facilitated our escape every time we walked through the park. But we never saw the feisty pooch again.

I learned a valuable life lesson from that experience: The best way to get out of trouble is to run. Get past it. Stay out of its reach.

That was my plan for cardiomyopathy. I'd outrun it, keep it behind me. Hopefully forever, but at least until my sons were adults and on their own. I chose to have those beautiful boys, and I would not mar their childhoods with fear and medical drama. It wasn't their fault I had some weird heart condition I couldn't even spell. My sons deserved carefree childhoods, and I would use every ounce of my strength to make sure they were childhoods that did not include worries about their mom's health.

As I lay in my hospital bed, an image of their sweet faces floated across my mind. Jeremy was sitting on the living room floor with Jonathan, surrounded by games, toys, and neighborhood boys. Out of nowhere, he stopped playing, looked around and said, "I love my life." The joy on his face, the pure contentment, took my breath away at the time. I didn't want anything, ever, to steal that happiness from his heart.

Once again, warrior mode kicked in. The same overwhelming protectiveness I felt at my sons' births invaded every cell in my body and filled me with resolve. Gerry and I would give our children happy childhoods and tuck my health drama away in a hidden corner of our marriage. I wasn't sure how, exactly, but it wasn't up for discussion. Regardless of what the doctors said, I would force my heart to keep beating.

CHAPTER FOUR:
YOU WANT TO DO WHAT?

For God is not a God of disorder but of peace.
(1 Corinthians 14:33)

I stayed in cardiac intensive care for a long time. My heart was dancing to a frenzied beat, and my body couldn't keep up. Dr. Strickman ordered a combination of drugs to strengthen my heart's pumping ability, stabilize its rhythm, and slow its rapid beat. Multiple IVs pumped diuretics into my veins to draw off excess fluid and ease the stress on my heart and kidneys.

While the medicine worked to strengthen my heart, Dr. Strickman talked with Gerry in the hallway outside my room. "You need to check with your insurance company to see if they will cover the cost of a heart transplant. We need to be prepared in case the medication proves ineffective."

Gerry nodded and told the doctor he'd check right away. But inside he was reeling. A heart transplant? Weren't they incredibly risky? The thought of raising two young boys on his own nearly paralyzed him. He retreated to a quiet corner of the waiting room to steady his nerves and pull his thoughts away from the yawning abyss of fear. Then he called our insurance company, grateful to have a concrete task to perform.

When Dr. Strickman shared the transplant idea with me, I tried to keep my face neutral, listen to the words coming out of his mouth, and not completely flip out. But it was nearly impossible to process those words. How could he suggest such a crazy, radical, violent act?

Then I thought about the young woman down the hall with cardiomyopathy. I'd asked my nurse about her earlier that morning and learned she had died during the night. It didn't seem right for me to dismiss the transplant idea out of hand when she had not been given the opportunity to choose.

The insurance company approved the procedure, so Dr. Strickman ordered a slew of additional tests to see if I was a candidate for transplantation. There is a severe shortage of available organs, and doctors do everything they can to make sure the rest of a person's body is healthy before they consider placement on the transplant list. I agreed to the testing because Dr. Strickman said it was necessary, but I did not believe anything would come of it. This heart business would prove to be a weird health glitch, a fluke. Regardless of what Houston's medical gurus said, my heart would get better and keep on ticking. I planned to go home, make a full recovery, and get on with the rest of my life.

Being separated from my children was the most difficult part of my time in intensive care. My husband was allowed to visit, but my children were too young to be allowed in my room. I went nuts worrying about them and missed their sweet faces with an ache far deeper than any caused by a bum heart. I missed snuggling with Jeremy and reading his favorite bedtime stories. I missed Jonathan's fierce hugs and peeling the skin off his hot dogs and apples.

"When can I see my children?" I asked my doctors and nurses. "I've never been away from them for this long. They won't understand why I'm not there." I pleaded with any medical professional unlucky enough to walk into my room. "Please, let me see my sons."

A few days later one of the nurses pushed a wheelchair into my room and began unplugging machines. "More tests?" I asked. "I thought we were done."

"No tests," she said and hooked the IVs to a battery pack. "I'm taking you to see your children."

Tears flowed down my cheeks as my kindhearted superhero nurse helped me put on a robe, comb my hair, and try to look less scary and more like the pre-hospital me. Then she arranged me in the wheelchair and rolled me to an empty conference room. "Thank you," I told her. "Thank you *so* much."

A few minutes later Gerry pushed the door open a crack and peeked into the room.

"Can we come in?" he asked.

"Yes!" I squealed.

Gerry opened the door wide and I saw them, Jeremy on one side of his dad, Jonathan on the other.

"Come in, come in," I said, smiling like Christmas morning. "It's so good to see you. You guys look great!" I flung my arms out wide, hoping they'd rush in for a hug. But Jonny kept his eyes on the floor and leaned against Gerry's side. Jeremy stared at the IV bags, shuffled from one foot to the other, and glanced at me a few times.

"It's okay," I said. "This medicine is making me feel better so I can come home. Don't worry, I'll be there before you know it." I acted happy and upbeat, babbled on and on, and tried to reassure them that everything was fine, fine, fine, and I'd be home soon.

No one bought what I was selling, and the visit ended a few minutes later. As soon as my family left, my cheery mom-mask crumbled, and I had my first major meltdown. It was obvious my children were scared and uncomfortable with the hospital sights and smells. Of course, it was scary for them—it was scary for me. I'd hoped seeing me would reassure them and show them I was okay, but I feared I'd made a bad situation worse. I realized asking my children to come to the hospital was an incredibly selfish act, a mistake I would not repeat. They'd see me at home, soon, when I looked and felt a bit more human.

Transplant evaluation testing finally ended. Dr. Strickman took my file to a transplant approval meeting, and I was approved and placed on the heart transplant waiting list. My position was nowhere near the top of the list, the spots reserved for the sickest patients. Dr. Strickman hoped my heart would stabilize and I could avoid a transplant. But he put me on the list in case that didn't happen.

Day by slow day, I grew stronger and felt more like myself. The water weight I'd gained fell off, and my heart and kidneys stabilized. I was moved out of intensive care and into a regular room where friends and family were now allowed to visit. I was still hooked up to lots of monitors, and Gerry watched the numbers on the machines slide up and down as people dropped in to offer encouragement.

My mom visited on the Fourth of July weekend. "There are a lot of car accidents on the Fourth of July," she said. "Maybe you'll get a heart this weekend." I know she was trying to reassure me I'd be home soon, but I had no words in response to her comment. I felt gutted. *No, I don't want anyone to die in a car wreck so I can get their heart. No!* When the numbers on my heart monitors zoomed upward and the machines began to beep and flash red, Gerry steered Mom out to the waiting room.

When friends stopped by, I was able to thank them for the many ways they had helped my family and me during my hospital incarceration. Ms. Pat, a dear friend and a retired nurse, came to our house every day and took care of Jeremy and Jonathan with grandmotherly devotion. She helped them draw pictures for Mommy, took them to the park, blew bubbles with their bubble wands, tossed balls, played games on the living room floor, and made life as normal as possible for them. She even kept a notebook for me and wrote down their daily activities so I could experience a small part of those missed days.

A kind hospital volunteer came to my room and washed my hair in the bed because I felt inhuman after being in the hospital for such a long time. I was in the hospital during Father's Day and wasn't able to buy Father's Day cards for the children to give to Gerry. A friend bought them for me and took them to the hospital so I could sign them for the boys.

One of the local churches sent over many days' worth of meals for Gerry and the boys. We'd never even attended that church. Friends and acquaintances put me on prayer chains all over the country. A local Christian radio station asked for prayers for me, and strangers popped in at the hospital and told me they were praying.

I appreciated the support but was skeptical about the prayers. For years, I had prayed and pleaded with God to heal my sister Chris's Crohn's disease. I'd cried buckets of tears, made deals, and bargained with God to end her suffering, but Crohn's disease continued to plague Chris's life. I did not understand how a loving God could allow an innocent young girl to suffer so horribly.

The Bible tells us to study God's word and pray. If we pray, he will listen. When Chris got sick, I read the Bible, researched, and studied, determined to keep at it until I found a logical explanation for my sister's suffering. I zeroed in on key verses like, "Ask and it will be given to you; seek and you will find; knock and the door will be opened to you" (Luke 11:9) and "And the prayer offered in faith will make the sick person well" (James 5:15). But Chris did not get well, and her illness convinced me that if God answered prayers, they were someone else's prayers. He was deaf to my pleas. Therefore, God was for other people, not me.

So, as I grappled with my own health crisis, I thanked the hospital visitors for their prayers and smiled politely, but I did not expect any divine intervention. If I was going to get well, I would rely on Dr. Strickman and the medicine he prescribed. I would follow his instructions faithfully, eat super healthy food, cut out all strenuous activity, and beat this heart thing on my own.

CHAPTER FIVE:
TREADING WATER

With man this is impossible, but with God all things are possible. (Matthew 19:26)

Dr. Strickman finally released me from the hospital. I was technically on the heart transplant list but near the bottom. If my heart continued to strengthen, Dr. Strickman would remove my name from the list. If things grew worse, he could easily increase my position. I felt confident that would not be necessary. I planned to be the poster child for healthy living.

With an armful of drugs, we headed home to find a new normal. One question flickered through my brain like an annoying gnat—was this a new beginning or the beginning of the end? My discharge instructions included a simple plan for a modified lifestyle: eat a low-salt diet and don't do anything that elevated my heart rate. That meant no exercise, no lifting anything heavier than a few pounds, and no work. The work ban was the hardest part of the plan to adhere to. I've worked since I was fifteen. I enjoy work. It's part of who I am.

Before I got sick, I owned and operated a computer training company. It was the perfect job for me at the time, a combination of my teaching background and the computer skills I'd acquired through the school of work-your-rear-off. The training center was close to home and I'd scheduled classes three days a week so I could be home with Jeremy and Jonathan the rest of the time. After a few weeks home from the hospital, I closed the training center, shut down the business, and found buyers for the computer equipment.

Caring for my family and performing everyday household tasks became hurdles to conquer. With the tiniest bit of exertion, I could feel my heart hammering in my chest. I had to do everything s-l-o-w-l-y, and for a born multitasker, used to zipping from one thing to another, it wasn't easy for me. I no longer pitched when Jeremy and Jonny played baseball in the cul-de-sac. I sat in a chair in the yard and cheered. I did household chores in shifts. Carry a few dirty clothes to the laundry room. Rest. Carry a few more. Rest. A few more. Rest. Load the washing machine. Rest. Dump a few wet clothes in the dryer. Rest. Dump a few more. Rest. Everything I did took forever, and patience has never been a quality I can claim.

Gerry stopped home for lunch one day and found me sitting on the living room floor.

"What are you doing?" he said, panic in his voice. "Are you okay?"

"I'm fine," I said and dragged myself up off the floor. "Just taking a little break."

A flock of friends helped ease me into my new role as a heart disease survivor. My friend Diane flew from Memphis to Houston to see me, even though she didn't have the money for a spontaneous trip. We hugged, we cried, and she listened to me vent without judgment. And as always, she made me laugh with her one-of-a-kind, quirky stories and lifted my spirits with an outpouring of love.

Sandy, a neighborhood friend, came over every Friday morning, drove me to the grocery store, pushed the cart, loaded the car, and unpacked the groceries in my kitchen. People I barely knew sent cards and notes of encouragement. Lots of people from churches in the area sent meals. A group of women cleaned our house.

With all that help and extra time on my hands, I attempted to become a better homemaker for my family. Housework was not a problem. I kept our home and clothing clean and neat, no problem. The problem was cooking. You'd think I would know how to cook, as I grew up in a big Italian Irish family in a suburb of Chicago. We lived near our paternal grandparents and visited them often. Frank Sr. grew tomatoes and grapes in a large garden beside their house and made wine in the basement. My grandmother, Agnes, made homemade bread, homemade pasta, and the best spaghetti sauce this side of Italy. As a child, I used to stare open-mouthed as she stuck her index finger and thumb into a boiling pot of spaghetti, pulled out a pale-yellow strand, and plopped it in her mouth to taste for doneness.

I did not inherit her cooking gene. In fact, I've always been a lousy cook, and the stuff I knew how to make was not particularly healthy. My friends stepped in once again and brought over several shiny hardback cookbooks with low-salt recipes. I studied those recipes, made tidy lists of ingredients for our shopping expeditions, and faithfully followed seemingly endless lines of instructions. But it was useless. No book, friendly encouragement, or health incentive could turn me into a good cook. I could do it for a few days. But every day? There were too many unread books waiting for me by my snuggly chair to waste time in the kitchen.

Doctors told me when I left the hospital it was rare for a heart as damaged as mine to repair itself to any significant degree. But slowly, month by month, my heart grew stronger. As my health improved, I eased back into the life I had before heart disease announced itself. Jeremy played soccer, and driving him to practice and watching his games felt like winning the lottery. Jonathan joined a T-ball team, his first experience with organized sports. At his first game, he stepped up to the T, looked at the ball, got ready to swing the bat, and then turned to find me in the stands. When he found me, he set the bat on the ground, and with a dramatic wave, blew me a kiss. Then he picked up the bat and hit the ball. I swallowed the lump in my throat, and a collective "Ahhhhh," went up from the stands as every mom around me melted into her seat.

My social circle expanded and dozens of people, both close friends and casual acquaintances, talked to me about God. They thought it was a miracle I was doing so well. They asked if I was on my knees constantly, thanking God for his blessings.

Nope, not really. I was busy trying to stay alive.

I followed Dr. Strickman's instructions to the letter and attributed my recovery to the cardiology team at St. Luke's Hospital and the scientists who developed the handfuls of drugs I took every day to keep my heart beating. But as the months passed, new questions and new ideas slowly seeped into my brain.

Doctors and scientists can't *make* my heart beat. Sure, they can use their brilliant minds and the scientific knowledge they've acquired through years of study to come up with a treatment plan. But they can't guarantee the results. They can't say *for sure* it will work for every patient.

I accepted the fact that I can't *make* my heart beat. Sure, I can faithfully take my medicine, watch my salt intake, and rest when my body needs it. I can avoid strenuous activities, live a sedentary lifestyle, and become the poster child for healthy living.

But I can't *make* my heart beat. I can't will myself to live.

A radical idea took hold: I am not in control. All the independence and self-sufficiency I thought I had was an illusion. No matter how hard I try, I can't will myself to live if it is time for me to die.

So, if I'm not in control, who is?

Sleep became an elusive stranger as I wrestled with questions swirling inside my brain. Is life a random series of events, simply the luck of the draw? Or do our life experiences have a purpose? I didn't believe we drifted through life dealing with whatever the cosmos threw our way, and then one day, died. Too many incredible, unexplainable things had happened in my life to believe it's all up to chance. Eluding the man in the park when I was a child, meeting Gerry in Monte's office for a project that didn't exist, and the unexpected phone call that led from Memphis to St. Louis to the birth of my children. Each of those events took on greater significance. Could they have been orchestrated by a higher power?

As my heart continued to repair itself and grow stronger, I had no answers for the cosmic questions that robbed my sleep at night. But they kept hammering away at me, demanding answers. So, Gerry, the boys, and I started attending church services. Maybe I'd find answers there.

CHAPTER SIX:
UNDERSTANDING DAWNS

Trust in the LORD with all your heart and lean not on your own understanding. (Proverbs 3:5)

Gerry and I began attending church services and Sunday school classes with Jeremy and Jonathan. I read the Bible on my own and slowly learned the story of God's love for us through Jesus. For the first time in my life, Jesus became more to me than stories in an old book. I saw how he is active in the world today and cares about our struggles—my personal struggles, my fears, and my doubts. It didn't happen overnight, but one by one, my questions fell away. I didn't have answers to all of them, didn't suddenly understand why Chris has a lousy gut or I have a bum ticker. But I realized I'm not meant to understand every single thing in the universe. I'm not God. I learned to say, "That's okay. I trust you, God," and mean it.

Even with faith, bad things happen. People get sick. Children die. Injustice flourishes. I accepted the fact that God is not a cosmic genie, although I had treated him like one my whole life. Being a Christian did not mean I could mumble a few prayers, and whoosh, God would grant my every desire. Sometimes his plan is not the same as my plan, and even though I ask through prayer, I may not get what I want.

I learned it's not about the size of my faith; it's about the *object* of my faith. God created the universe. He has THE plan, and his plan is perfect. As the master creator, the designer of the universe, he is not obligated to share the details with me.

God had finally gotten my attention. I saw my heart was damaged spiritually as well as physically. If doctors fixed the physical problem, it meant nothing if I didn't fix the spiritual problem. Whether I died today or fifty years from now, death was in my future. Where I choose to spend eternity is the most important decision I will make in this brief life.

I accepted Jesus as my personal savior and Lord and became a Christian. Since God determined when I was born and when I will die, I stopped agonizing over what I had done to cause heart disease. I quit worrying about whether I was doing enough to help my body heal. Secure in the knowledge God has a plan for my life, I plugged into life with a stronger current and looked for ways to complete whatever he wanted me to accomplish in this life.

As a new believer struggling with chronic illness, I had to depend on God daily as I adjusted to a modified lifestyle and a regimen of limited activity, doctor's appointments, and the side effects of lots of medication. I focused on my family and became intentional about showing my love for them each day, through words and actions. It wasn't always easy.

When Jeremy turned seven, Gerry decided he was old enough to own his first knife.

"No, absolutely not, he's too young," I said.

"I got my first knife when I was five," Gerry said. "Every boy needs a knife. I'll teach him how to use it safely."

"A little boy does not *need* a knife. He'll hurt himself. Please, don't buy him a knife."

I lost the argument, and Gerry bought Jeremy a knife.

At his birthday party, Jeremy and his buddies ate burgers and hot dogs, played games, and enjoyed cake and ice cream. The house vibrated with the glorious sound of laughing boys. Jeremy opened his gifts and was thrilled with his new knife. Gerry cautioned him the knife was not a toy and showed him which side of the blade was sharp. He showed him how to open and close the knife safely and had Jeremy practice a few times in front of us. Then the boys scampered off to the playroom.

We heard the screams a few minutes later.

Gerry and I raced to the playroom and found Jeremy holding his hand. Blood dripped through his fingers, onto his jeans, and pooled in the carpet.

"Grab a towel," Gerry said.

He wrapped Jeremy's finger with the towel and held it tight to stop the bleeding. I ran to the bathroom for bandages. By the time I got back to the playroom with the bandages, the towel around Jeremy's finger was red, soaked with my precious son's blood.

"He's going to need stitches," Gerry said.

At that moment I was so angry, I thought my head would explode. I had never, not once in my entire life, felt such overwhelming rage at another human being. I couldn't look at Gerry. *Why did he have to buy the stupid knife?*

We loaded Jeremy's friends into our van and dropped them off on our way to the emergency room. Then the four of us huddled in a cubicle at the hospital and tried to console Jeremy while doctors assessed the cut on his finger.

Jeremy's screams filled the emergency room corridor, and one of the nurses closed the door to our tiny compartment to cut down on the general bedlam. Unfortunately, she shut the heavy hospital door on two of Jonathan's fingers.

The chaos level doubled when Jon began howling and his fingers turned black. Gerry took Jonathan to be treated in another cubicle, and I stood beside Jeremy and held his good hand while a doctor sewed seven stitches into his tiny finger. Both of our sons were now bandaged and broken on a day that was meant to be a happy, carefree birthday celebration.

I could not forgive Gerry. I blamed him for injuring our children. The Bible says we need to forgive others as Christ forgave us, but I couldn't do it. I knew Jeremy and Jonathan would both be fine. Their fingers would heal. But the entire episode was unnecessary. If Gerry had listened to me when I pleaded with him to wait a few years on the knife idea, Jeremy and Jonny would not have suffered unnecessary, pointless pain.

Gerry did not understand my rage. "Jeremy knows how to close a knife now," he said.

That put me over the top. The incident became symbolic of an imbalance in our marriage where Gerry made all the decisions and my opinion was not considered. We'd have to divorce—there was no way I could live with *that person*. Jeremy and Jonny would be split between households. They'd be traumatized, maybe for life, have to undergo years of counseling, never find wives, never know the joy of a happy marriage. My mind spiraled down a dark rabbit hole of bleak futures for all of us.

Then I started to pray. I admitted to God I was incapable of forgiving my husband. I asked him to show me a way to let go of the anger that coursed through my veins like molten lava. I prayed every day. I prayed every night. I prayed a lot.

After a while, I realized I could look at Gerry without wanting to punch him in the face. My anger was gone. God had answered my prayers.

I also realized being a Christian did not mean life would always be sparkly princess dances on puffy clouds. I still had heart disease. I still fought with my husband. Life was hard. But with God at the center of my life, I slowly learned to put life's challenges in their proper place—temporary, fleeting struggles when compared to the eternity awaiting us with Christ in heaven.

Jeremy and Jonathan were now in school all day, and I found myself with hours of empty time. I couldn't do the work I had done before cardiomyopathy. Anything that elevated my heart rate was off limits. I needed to find a useful way to fill my days, and I wanted it to be more than a job. I wanted to find a meaningful new career, one that contributed to the world in a positive way. It had to be a sedentary occupation and one that involved children. What could I do from home, sitting, that involved children in some way?

God provided the perfect solution: writing children's books. I love reading and learning about new things—why not combine my two great loves, children and books?

I didn't know the first thing about how to write a children's book. So, I took a correspondence course in creative writing from my alma mater, the University of Texas at Austin. This was pre-internet, so the UT professor sent a packet with instructions for the first lesson, and I mailed my typed responses back to him. The professor graded it and sent it back to me along with the next lesson. I learned a ton in that class and discovered I enjoyed the challenge of finding the best combination of words to precisely express an idea. I had never thought about how a single word can change the tone of a piece of writing. It was fascinating, and I was hooked.

I joined the Society of Children's Book Writers and Illustrators and attended conferences and workshops to learn about the craft of writing as well as tips on how to break into the business. Children's book writers are a wonderful tribe—open, funny, big-hearted, helpful, and really smart. I soaked up their wisdom like a sponge. At my first writers' conference, I won an award for the first five pages of my novel-in-progress. As a result of that award, a lovely and brilliant children's author with more than one hundred books in print mentored me for a year. I met with her at her home in Houston and spent hours discussing my manuscript and the business of writing for children.

What a confidence boost!

I finished the novel and submitted it to literary agents and publishers. It was rejected by one and all. Seasoned writers encourage new writers to write what they know, so I tried a different approach—writing nonfiction instead of fiction. In the early years of our marriage, I had worked as a computer programmer for several large corporations. So, I combined my computer knowledge with my teaching experience and wrote a computer programming book for young adults. It sold, along with a similar book in a different computer programming language.

Gerry and I flew to the East Coast for a book signing tour when the books were released. We had a blast visiting my sister Kathy and her family, zipping from bookstore to bookstore, chatting with customers about writing, and signing books. But the demand for computer programming books for children was not exactly fever pitch. After the first burst of excitement at holding books with my name on the cover, life settled back into its regular rhythms. And I went back to sitting at my computer for hours each day, staring at the screen, and searching for the right combination of words to bring a story to life.

I rewrote my novel, and the new version was also rejected by publishers. I wrote a new novel, this one about a teenage computer hacker. It won a writing contest too, and I found a literary agent who agreed to represent me. But that book didn't sell either. I studied the craft of writing, read a ton of how-to books by successful authors, and attended writing conferences and workshops in Houston, Dallas, and Austin. I took classes, entered contests, and joined a critique group. And I wrote. A lot. But all my manuscripts were rejected by publishers and literary agents.

Discouragement replaced the heady excitement of creating something unique. I started to doubt—maybe writing wasn't God's plan for me. Maybe I was a talentless hack masquerading as a writer. But I kept working, kept studying, and kept learning. Through a writers' newsletter, I saw an article about a nonfiction publisher looking for writers for a series of American history books for children.

Perfect, I thought. *I love history!*

All I had to do to land the job was figure out how to write a book proposal.

CHAPTER SEVEN:
A NEW LIFESTYLE

Let us run with perseverance the race marked out for us.
(Hebrews 12:1)

Seasoned writers advise newbies-with-a-dream to follow publisher guidelines to the letter when writing a book proposal. I worked on a writing sample for the American history series, studied books published by the publishing company, and agonized over a cover letter that wouldn't make me sound like a complete rookie. Then I sent the publisher a proposal and crossed my fingers. A couple of months later, shock of all shocks, they offered me a book contract. Whoo-hoo! Dancing in the street time!

The book they hired me to write was a creative nonfiction title about Hull-House, a settlement house in Chicago set in 1908. Hull-House is now a National Historic Landmark and a Chicago Landmark, which made research a lot of fun. I flew to Chicago, toured the Hull-House Museum, and spent long days at the University of Illinois at Chicago doing research.

It was great to be back in Chicago. I splurged and stayed at the famous Palmer House hotel. Each morning, armed with notebooks, pencils, and pens, I headed to the U of I campus, plopped down at a table in the research department, and read hundreds of letters handwritten more than one hundred years ago by the founder of Hull-House, Jane Addams. I studied countless period newspaper articles and telegrams and took notes until my fingers cramped. Each time I uncovered an interesting tidbit, my excitement grew. I wanted to share all the cool stuff I discovered with the world.

I learned a ton about writing books, editing, and the publishing process on that project. Research became my passion. With so many amazing stories to uncover, researching a book morphed into the greatest treasure hunt ever. After *Hull-House* was released, nonfiction publishers offered me biographies and American histories to write. I didn't make a lot of money, but I had steady, interesting work.

Biographies were fun to write. I enjoyed getting to know my subjects and tried to decipher the whys in their lives as well as the whats. When I researched Andrew Carnegie's life for a young adult biography, I flew to Washington, DC, and found letters at the Library of Congress he'd written to presidents Grover Cleveland, William McKinley, Theodore Roosevelt, and William Taft. In the handwritten letters, Carnegie offered his advice and recommendations on how to handle the crisis of the moment. Mark Twain's letters to Carnegie were my favorites, his wit on full display, even in his personal correspondence. I felt like I'd lucked into the coolest job in the world—getting paid to learn fascinating stuff about awesome people and write about it for children.

Shortly after the September 11 terrorist attacks in 2001, one of my publishers hired me to write a biography of First Lady Laura Bush. At the time, President George W. Bush's approval rating was 90 percent. Most Americans agreed with the way he was handling the aftermath of the terrorist attacks.

As I researched her life, I grew to admire Laura Bush and found lots of similarities between us. She had attended my alma mater, the University of Texas at Austin, and was a book lover, an avid reader, and a teacher. She seemed like someone I could easily be friends with, which made her biography a pleasure to write. Unfortunately, by the time the book was released, President Bush's approval rating had plunged to 31 percent. He no longer had the support of the American people. My Laura Bush biography sold few copies and was taken out of circulation quickly.

In spite of the ups and downs of book sales, writing turned out to be the best possible job for a mom with young children and heart disease. I doubt I would have attempted it if cardiomyopathy hadn't chained me to a desk. But since it was a chain God designed for me, I fell in love with my new career and felt blessed to have found a sedentary job with beauty and purpose.

The best part of my new lifestyle? I could turn off my computer when Jeremy and Jonathan came home from school and spend time with my precious sons. I could also drive them to soccer practice, basketball practice, guitar lessons, piano lessons, viola lessons, and lots and lots of games. We didn't talk about cardiomyopathy, and they didn't know about the handful of pills I took each day to keep my heart beating. Life settled into a regular routine, and heart disease faded into the background.

I checked in with Dr. Strickman every six months, then once a year. He'd run tests, tweak my medications, and send me on my way until the next year. It was inconvenient to drive to his office at the huge medical center in downtown

Houston. Traffic was grueling and each appointment ate up an entire day. But it became a vital thread in the fabric of our lives.

Before Gerry and I could blink, Jeremy and Jonathan started high school. They both became Christians and were active in church youth group activities. Jeremy played guitar and led his school worship band, earned a black belt in tae kwon do, and played on the soccer team. Jonathan played viola in the school orchestra and played on the basketball and soccer teams. They started driving, which gave them a lot more independence and ushered in a whole new set of challenges.

My dad used to tell me I had a "heavy foot" when I was a teenager, and he repeatedly cautioned me to slow down when I was behind a steering wheel. He was right. I got my first speeding ticket when I was sixteen years old, joyriding with my girlfriends. I hate to admit, it was the first of many speeding tickets I received as a teen and young adult. Both of my sons inherited my heavy foot, and paying for speeding tickets, driving them to the courthouse in downtown Houston traffic, and many, many driver education classes was more than enough payback for what I had put my parents through.

Jeremy and Jonathan may have had heavy feet as teenagers, but they also had kind, loving hearts. They spent part of each summer on mission trips serving others. On one trip, we flew to Racine, Wisconsin, and repaired houses in underprivileged neighborhoods. Since Gerry was a civil/structural engineer, he became a team leader and helped plan and oversee construction. I chaperoned the girls and slept on the floor with them in an old school. We worked hard, stayed hot and sweaty all the time, and didn't sleep much. But we felt a sense of accomplishment at seeing how the small improvements in their homes brought joy to the homeowners' lives. The trip held special significance for me because my heart had defied the odds and allowed me to share the experience with my sons.

Near the end of the weeklong trip, each team of volunteers was given a free afternoon to relax and recharge. It was the Fourth of July weekend, and Gerry and I wanted to do something special for our group. The teens had dedicated a week of their summer vacation to serve others, and they had done so with smiles on their faces and love in their hearts. I called my sister Kathy who lived about an hour away in Lake Forest, Illinois, at the time, and asked if we could use her pool and game room for a few hours.

"Sure, how many kids do you have with you?" Kathy asked.

"Eighteen, but don't worry. They're great kids."

"I'm not worried. See you soon."

In the time it took for us to drive from Racine, Wisconsin, to Lake Forest, Illinois, Kathy and her husband Chad had made and bought a ton of food, set up festive tables and decorations around their pool, had music playing in the game room, and purchased a huge red, white, and blue cake. The teenagers had a fabulous time swimming and lounging in the pool, munching on snacks, playing pinball and foosball, and unwinding after a week of hard work. Gerry and I enjoyed our time catching up with Kathy and Chad, and the afternoon was a total win for the reenergized team of volunteers.

A few years later, Jeremy and then Jonny headed off to college. They both chose Texas schools, but paying for two overlapping college educations proved challenging. Gerry's engineering company had to cover the expense of an office, insurance, equipment, and employees, and some years were more profitable than others. My writing contracts provided steady work but not a lot of money. We wanted our sons to be debt free when they finished their educations, so to supplement the income I received from book royalties, I returned to teaching. I taught reading, language arts, and writing, first at a community college near my home and then at a private Christian school. My heart cooperated and allowed me the joy of helping financially support my children as they reached their educational goals.

Every so often, my heart flipped out and forgot how to pump strongly enough to move blood through my body. Sometimes it beat too fast, and sometimes it picked up a crazy rhythm. Then my kidneys would struggle, I'd retain water like crazy and gain a bunch of weight. When that happened, Dr. Strickman tweaked my prescriptions—a few more milligrams of this, a few less of that—and whipped my heart back into shape.

Or almost into shape. Each episode further weakened the weary muscle. I downplayed how tired I sometimes felt, kept smiling, and faked it. It was a technique I'd learned years earlier at a Fred Astaire Dance Studio in Houston.

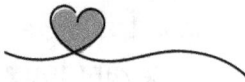

The year before I met Gerry, my friend Frances and I taught middle school together. She shared the most amazing stories of her worldwide travels. Many of her relatives lived in Greece, and Frances visited them often. She'd been to a slew of fascinating places in Europe, places I'd only dreamed about, as well as lots of other scenic destinations around the globe.

The year we taught together, the American Institute For Foreign Study sent a brochure to our school inviting teachers to participate in a summer foreign study program in Europe. The group of educators from the United States would study the educational systems of four European countries and compare them with the American educational system. Before I met Frances, I would have tossed the flyer in the trash. Post-Frances-friendship, I desperately wanted to go and see the things she so vividly described.

There was a problem, however—money. How in the world would I pay for a summer in Europe? At the time, I was an unmarried teacher living in a one-bedroom apartment so small I could stretch out my arms and practically touch the opposite living room walls. I had no savings account and little extra money. I took a part-time job to supplement my teacher's salary in hopes of earning enough for the trip. The job was doing simple bookkeeping for a small business. It was convenient, because I could work evenings and weekends. But I didn't earn enough to cover the expense of a summer in Europe. I needed a third job.

Between teaching and bookkeeping, my days were full. A third job would eat up every bit of my remaining free time, which I didn't mind if it got me to Europe. But I wanted the work to be something I enjoyed, a job where I could earn the money I needed for the trip and also have a bit of fun.

I love to dance and had danced in high school and college in musicals and with several dance troupes. I also love watching any kind of dance performance, so I thought it would be fun to hang out with dancers and work at a dance studio. Maybe I could answer phones, schedule appointments, or do bookkeeping. I drove around Houston and found a Fred Astaire Dance Studio not far from my apartment. I barged in one afternoon without an appointment and asked if they needed any help. The manager put on some music, twirled me around the studio for a while, and hired me.

As a dance instructor? Oh dear, I think I'm in over my head.

Since I didn't know the first thing about ballroom dancing, the manager gave me a thick three-ring binder with all the dances the studio taught. Each dance had a series of small footprints that showed the steps and the rhythm of the dance. I studied that binder and came to work early each day so seasoned instructors could somehow turn me into a ballroom dancer.

It wasn't easy for them. I didn't have enough time to memorize all the steps to all the dances, so I did the best I could with my limited skills. Once, when I was teaching the tango to a young couple, I didn't know enough tango steps to fill the hour-long lesson. So, I made up steps. I figured the students were there to have fun, to move, to dance. Dancing wasn't about matching the little footprints in my Fred Astaire binder. It was about music and movement and joy. The students didn't know the steps they learned that day weren't official steps in my Fred Astaire binder. But they were happy as pumpkin pie—they were dancing!

The studio manager stood nearby watching the lesson, and he did not look happy.

After the clients left, the manager called me into his office and closed the door. I thought I was about to lose my job. "You know that wasn't a tango you were teaching back there," he said.

I nodded, embarrassed that my pitiful sham as a dance instructor had been revealed. In my mind's eye, I watched my summer in Europe evaporate like early morning mist on the ocean I'd never cross.

Then the manager surprised me, grinned, and said, "You may not know how to dance, but as long as the customers are happy, I'm happy."

Wait, I'm not fired?

"Try and learn a few more steps," he added.

I sagged in my chair with relief. "Yes, sir."

Every Thursday evening, students and instructors attended a studio-wide dance. Students could dance with different instructors or with different student partners. Instructors demonstrated dances during breaks. The first time I had to demonstrate a dance, one of the seasoned instructors told me to smile, follow him, and no matter what happened, keep dancing.

I learned more than ballroom dancing at Fred Astaire. I learned that sometimes in life, you have to let go of control and rely on experts to pull you through. My fellow instructors pulled me through at Fred Astaire, and my students never suspected I was a rookie masquerading as a dance instructor. The money I earned at the studio allowed me to spend a glorious summer in London, Paris, Rome, and Athens.

The same technique worked for years with cardiomyopathy. Dr. Strickman and his team of experts pulled me through years of heart disease. I was able to watch my children grow into independent adults, oblivious of my heart condition. And Gerry and I kept dancing through the years.

CHAPTER EIGHT:
IT'S ALWAYS SOMETHING

God is our refuge and strength, an ever-present help in trouble. (Psalm 46:1)

Year after year, my heart chugged along. Jeremy and Jon finished their educations and launched careers. I began traveling again and took a trip to Tuscany, Italy, with two dear friends. We stayed in an ancient convent with exposed stonework, beamed ceilings, and a few scorpions I pretended not to see.

Our days began at the piazza in Cortona, the City of Art. We sipped cappuccino, nibbled biscotti or freshly baked bread with jam, and watched the medieval town come to life. Then we drove from one ancient hamlet to the next, past fertile valleys filled with olives, fruit orchards, or wine vineyards. I learned a whole new set of driving rules in Rome. A green light means GO! GO! GO! A red light is just a suggestion. And a yellow light? Yellow is for gaiety, no need to slow down. Other driving tips I picked up in Italy: Lanes? Variety is the spice of life—try them all. Speed limits? The faster the better. Parking? If you see an inch of space, go for it!

We walked for hours each day and explored castles and cathedrals. We saw Renaissance frescoes and priceless art in Siena, San Gimignano, and Montepulciano. In Florence, we went on a Michelangelo pilgrimage and were awed by the beauty and lifelike energy of his sculptures.

And we ate the most delicious food in the world.

"Spaghetti? Again?" said my friend Linda as we lounged over our afternoon splurge meal. "You need to try something different. Expand your horizons."

"This is different," I said and savored another scrumptious bite. "And it's definitely expanding all of my horizons. I had no idea there were so many types of sauces for spaghetti. I want to try every one of them."

When our feet gave out at the end of each day, and we couldn't take another step, we ate gelato under the bright Tuscan sun. I enjoyed every second of that once-in-a-lifetime trip, even more so because heart disease had faded into the background and no longer held center stage in my life. As long as I tossed down a handful of pills each morning, I was good to go.

Life is a combination of joy and sorrow, and every family experiences sadness and loss. My family was no exception. My younger brother Michael had suffered from severe back pain for years. He refused to consider back surgery and relied on pain medication and alcohol to get him through his days. Two failed marriages left him devastated, and combined with constant pain, plunged him into a deep depression. He talked about ending his life.

I felt like I was standing in the path of a speeding train, waving my arms over my head in a frantic attempt to stop a catastrophe. I called the suicide hotline and talked with counselors about how to help my brother. I tried to pull him out of his depression and show him how much he was loved. We traveled to California together to visit our mom and went to Dallas to see Chris. I popped over to his house as often as possible to provide a listening ear. I talked to him about God's love for him, shared the gospel, and invited him to our church. Michael and Gerry shared a love of Harley Davidson motorcycles, and Gerry reached out to him, rode with him, and talked with him for hours about all things Harley.

But our love for Michael couldn't save him. One cold night in December, he dialed 911 and told the dispatcher he was going to commit suicide. Then he pulled out a gun and shot himself. As he lived alone, I guess he wanted to make sure his body was found. I was brokenhearted by his decision to end his life and furious at the same time. My sister Chris and I had both fought through years of pain and kept going. Medical advances took place all the time. Maybe there was a doctor somewhere who could fix Michael's back. Why didn't he find that doctor? Why didn't he ask God for the strength to fight? But after the anger drained away, I realized I didn't walk in his shoes and didn't understand the depths of his despair. I was left with a deep, profound sadness I knew would always be a part of me.

Joy followed sorrow, as it always does. Jeremy met a lovely woman named Colleen. They married and moved to St. Louis, Missouri, where Colleen began her residency in pediatric medicine and Jeremy worked as a counseling intern. Jon, the technical guru of the family, lived in downtown Houston. He worked for a large corporation and did something complicated with computers. God had answered my prayers and allowed me the privilege of watching my sons blossom into incredible young men.

A few months after Jeremy's wedding, my heart flipped out again. I couldn't catch my breath, my kidneys grew sluggish, and I gained a ton of weight. I pretended I was fine and hoped that if I kept going, I would be. But the plan didn't work. As days turned into a week, then two, simple everyday tasks became challenges. I needed to rest after walking across a room, coughed my head off, and couldn't sleep. Dr. Strickman increased the dosage on my meds, and I tried that for several weeks. It didn't help. He ordered blood work and an echocardiogram in his office. Then he ordered a stress test.

I'd had lots of heart tests through the years, but I'd never had a stress test. Dr. Strickman wanted to watch how my heart reacted when I exercised. One of his nurses led me to a room in his office complex with a fancy treadmill, and technicians hooked me up to a bunch of monitors. Although I hadn't walked on a treadmill in years, I felt confident I could walk for a good long while. After all, five years earlier I had traipsed around Tuscany without a single heart problem.

Dr. Strickman stood nearby, his eyes on the computer screen monitoring my heart, and I began to walk. I'd barely gotten started when he stopped the test.

"That's enough," he said and turned off the treadmill. "I've seen what I needed to see."

I was confused. It had taken the technicians longer to hook up all the wires on my chest than I'd walked on the treadmill. How could he tell anything about my heart with such a short test?

"You need to be in the hospital," said Dr. Strickman.

"Why? What did the test show?"

"We need to run more tests," he said. "But it looks like your heart has deteriorated somewhat. We'll know more after we run additional tests."

"When do you want me to go?"

"Right now. Is your husband with you?"

I nodded. "He's in the waiting room."

"I'll go talk to him, and my nurse will call the hospital and tell them you're on your way. I'll check in on you later tonight."

I DID NOT want to go to the hospital. I know they're wonderful places where brilliant doctors work miracles and save lives. But I did not want to be one of them. I wanted Dr. Strickman to hand me some new miracle pills and get my heart working again. I wanted to go home and continue my quiet life with my husband. I wanted to read books, write books, and spend time with my family and friends. Lying in a hospital bed was not on my agenda.

"I haven't been in a hospital in twenty years," I told Gerry as he drove to St. Luke's.

"That's true," he said, "but Dr. Strickman doesn't mess around. He'll fix you up and get you out of there in no time."

My eyes filled with tears. "I know, but that's not what I meant," I said. "For years, I've been praying and asking God to keep me alive long enough to raise our children. Jeremy just got married, and Jonny is thriving on his own with a great job and a huge circle of friends. God answered my prayers."

Gerry glanced over at me and nodded. "You're right," he said. "God has blessed us in so many ways."

"Even though the hospital is the last place I want to go, don't you think the timing is incredible? Or should I say, divinely inspired? My heart didn't worsen until Jeremy and Jonathan were established in their careers and autonomous. Obviously, I don't want to deal with another bout of heart disease, but that was exactly what I prayed for."

I closed my eyes and thanked God for his faithfulness. Gerry reached over, squeezed my hand, and silently gave me the courage to take the next steps on my journey to heart health.

The hospital staff jumped into high gear when we got there. Nurses hung bags and bags of IVs and doctors ran lots of tests. I sat propped up in bed with a bunch of pillows, coughed, and tried not to pester my doctors about sending me home. Dr. Strickman is not only a brilliant cardiologist, he's also an exceptional human being, full of kindness and compassion. When the test results came in, he broke the bad news in the gentlest way possible.

"Your heart is not pumping well," he said. "The ejection fraction has decreased significantly."

I knew my ejection fraction, a measurement of how much blood the left ventricle pumps out with each contraction, was really low when I first learned I had heart disease. But it had improved over the years.

"Can you tell why it's gotten worse? It's been good for a long time."

"That's the nature of the disease," Dr. Strickman said. "The left ventricle, the main pumping chamber, is stretched out, too large to pump blood effectively through your body."

That doesn't sound good.

"In addition," he continued, "your aortic valve leaks, which over time, has damaged the area around it, the aortic root."

So, I have a fat, flabby heart that is stretched out like a worn-out balloon and leaks.

"How do we fix it?" I asked.

"You need a new aortic valve," Dr. Strickman said.

"You mean surgery?"

"Yes. We need to replace the valve. It will make you feel much better."

Dr. Strickman briefly outlined the surgery. There was a new technique where heart valves can be replaced without opening the chest. But that was not an option in my case because there was so much damage to the area around the valve. It would have to be open heart surgery, the one with a big incision down the chest, pulled open ribs, and a long recovery.

Bummer.

At fifty-nine years old, I'd never had surgery, and this one sounded like a doozy.

Did someone suck all the air out of the room?

"Is there anything else we can try to avoid surgery?" I asked Dr. Strickman.

"We've already tried it," he said.

I swallowed my fear and took a deep breath. If surgery was the only road home, then I'd force myself to do it. What choice did I have?

But there was another problem.

"The tests also revealed a spot on your left kidney," Dr. Strickman said.

"What does that mean?"

"You need to see a kidney specialist and have it checked out before we do the valve replacement surgery."

"What do you think it is?" I asked.

"It could be a benign cyst or it could be cancer."

"What does it look like to you?"

"It looks like cancer."

Dr. Strickman had already told Gerry about the possible cancer, and I guess they both expected me to flip out at the mention of the C word. I probably should have shown more emotion, but I figured it must not be too serious because I wasn't in pain. And even if it was cancer, I didn't see it as a death sentence. After all, heart disease is the leading cause of death worldwide and I'd been living with cardiomyopathy for twenty years. Cyst or cancer, it was merely another mountain to climb on the road home. Cut it out and let's get on with it. My goal was to endure whatever it took to fix what was broken and get back to life.

Dr. Strickman laid out a plan. Fix the kidney, and then, he'd find a surgeon to fix the heart valve. Since he was a cardiologist, not a surgeon, he promised to find the best valve surgeon in Houston for us.

But first, I had to find a kidney specialist.

CHAPTER NINE:
THE YEAR OF THE SCAR

My flesh and my heart may fail, but God is the strength of my heart and my portion forever. (Psalm 73:26)

I left the hospital with a sack of prescriptions and made an appointment to check out the spot on my kidney with Dr. Mark Sutton, a urologist. He ran his own tests and agreed with Dr. Strickman—probably cancer. He showed Gerry and me the scans and pointed out the location of the tumor. Its placement made it a possible candidate for a new procedure, one that used robot arms and small incisions to remove small kidney tumors.

Dr. Sutton referred us to Dr. Alvin Goh, the surgeon who had developed the new surgical technique. We met with him, and he ran additional tests and agreed to work with Dr. Sutton to remove the tumor. A few weeks later, Dr. Sutton and Dr. Goh performed robotic laparoscopic surgery and removed a section of my left kidney.

It was a brilliant technique. Several small slits in my back, abdomen, and side somehow allowed surgeons to control robot arms and pull out the cancer without the large incision kidney surgery typically requires. The cancer was small, stage 2, which meant it hadn't spread, and I still had most of my kidney. Recovery was quick since I didn't have a big incision to deal with. I was ready to move on to the heart valve problem.

A month after kidney surgery, I checked into the hospital to get a new and improved aortic valve. Dr. Strickman had found the top valve surgeon in Houston, and he agreed to do the surgery. Heart valves can be mechanical or animal, typically cow or pig valves. Dr. Ross Reul, my new heart surgeon, described each type and left Gerry and me to decide which one we wanted him to use.

"Which is worse," I asked my husband, "having part of a cow or pig in my chest, or a machine?"

Gerry ignored the question and focused on the pros and cons. "With an animal valve, you won't have to be on blood thinners," he said. "You won't have to do blood tests all the time."

"True," I agreed. "But animal valves wear out and need to be replaced every ten years."

He nodded. "That's the average. Maybe yours would last longer."

"I'm not sure I want to take that chance." As I pondered a question with no right answer I added, "Machines can have glitches and break. What if I get a wonky machine?"

"I'm not worried about the machine," said Gerry. "I'm sure it's fine. But can you handle needle sticks and blood tests for the rest of your life?"

I shrugged. "Is there an option C?"

This was a big surgery—open heart. The surgery where doctors cut open the chest and leave a huge, ugly, disgusting scar. Dr. Strickman assured us the surgery was *absolutely* necessary, no matter how many times I asked if he was sure he was sure. And there was no option C.

I chose a mechanical valve because I didn't want to take the chance an animal valve would wear out, and I'd need to repeat the surgery sometime in the future. One open heart surgery would definitely be enough, thank you very much.

Dr. Reul took out my aortic valve and replaced it with a mechanical valve. Then he removed the damaged section of my aorta and replaced it with an artificial tube. The procedure went well, there were no complications, and I was sent to cardiac ICU to recover.

The hospital had recently installed a new computer system for patient records, and nurses were unfamiliar with the software. When I woke up from surgery, I felt nauseous. I could see a group of nurses across the room working at their computer stations, but I could not get their attention because I was hooked up to a ventilator with my arms tied to the bed to prevent me from ripping it out. I lifted my head, wiggled from side to side, and moved as much as possible to get their attention. I tried to make some kind of noise. But their focus was totally riveted on the new computer software, and I was invisible.

It was a horrible feeling, trapped with my arms tied down and no way to communicate. I started to panic, and the nausea grew worse. *If I vomit in the breathing tube, I'll suffocate. No one will know until it's too late. All this for nothing.*

Finally, one of the nurses turned slightly, noticed I was awake, and came over to my bed. Just as I threw up in the tube.

That got her attention. She yanked out the tube, gave me some nausea medicine, and everything was fine. I didn't enjoy the yanking out part but was so relieved to have the breathing tube out and my arms free, it was worth it.

As I healed in the hospital, I let my doctors know at every opportunity I was ready to complete my recovery at home. As soon as possible. Or sooner.

"Part of the post-surgery protocol for mechanical valves involves daily doses of blood thinners," one of my doctors explained. "You need to be in the hospital because these blood thinners are given through IVs. We're monitoring your INR levels, or the amount of time it takes for your blood to clot, and when you get to the right level, you'll be able to go home."

"I've been on blood thinners before," I told him. "Dr. Strickman always gave them to me in pill form. And I have a blood testing machine at home, so I know how to measure my INR level."

"You will eventually take a prescription blood thinner and monitor your INR at home," the doctor said. "But right now, you need a stronger dosage, and this type of medicine doesn't come in pill form. In order for you to go home, someone would need to give you twice-daily shots in your abdomen to replace the medicine you're getting in the IVs."

Gerry and I looked at each other.

"Can you handle that?" I asked.

"Can you?"

"I'll close my eyes," I said. "The question is—can you stick me in the stomach with a needle twice a day?"

"I can if I have to."

I smiled at my sweet husband. "You have to."

We were out of that hospital as soon as the discharge papers were signed. Gerry became a pro at giving stomach shots, and my blood thinned enough to keep my new valve happy. It took about three months for my ribs and sternum to heal. I slowly got my strength back and rejoined the land of the healthy.

I had tons of energy with my new-and-improved-non-leaky valve and felt blessed that both the kidney surgery and the valve surgery were behind me. I went back to work writing books and teaching middle school language arts. I joined a line dance class, a tap dance class, and volunteered in a prison ministry that connected incarcerated mothers with their children through books. I became active in church ministries and spent as much time as possible with family and friends. I was back!

More focused than before the surgeries, I searched for purpose as each new day unfolded. Was there something God wanted me to do? A task I was too obtuse to acknowledge? I concentrated on my family and looked for ways to support and encourage each of them. I reached out to old friends and forged new friendships. The scar on my chest became a vivid reminder of God's blessings. Even though I didn't deserve it, even though I didn't understand why, God chose to keep me alive. I felt humbled and so, so grateful.

As I savored good health, life coasted along for several months.

Then Gerry got sick.

He had struggled with abdominal pain for months, but because of my health drama, he had ignored it.

"It feels like the same kind of pain I had before I had my gallbladder removed," he said.

"But you don't have a gallbladder anymore, so it can't be that," I said. "I don't have a clue, an ulcer, maybe?"

"I don't know, but I need to get rid of this pain in my gut."

Gerry made appointments with his gastroenterologist and his urologist. They each ran a bunch of tests and discovered a huge tumor on his right kidney.

The doctors agreed—it looked like cancer. Since the tumor was large, they felt the best solution would be to remove the entire kidney to prevent the cancer from spreading. Once again, we headed to the hospital, this time with Gerry as the patient and me as the trusted sidekick.

Dr. Sutton removed Gerry's right kidney laparoscopically. The surgery went well, and although the cancer was stage 3, there were no signs of disease outside the kidney. We were thrilled his doctors had found the cancer before it spread throughout his body. Another huge blessing was that Gerry did not need to have chemotherapy or radiation because the cancer was contained. The doctors felt confident they had removed all traces of the disease from his body. Gerry went home, healed, and slowly returned to his engineering work.

I thought kidney cancer showing up in both of us at the same time was odd. So, I racked my brain for bad habits that may have caused the disease to appear. We live a healthy lifestyle. The only possible villain I could see was our frequent cooking on a charcoal grill. I had no scientific proof to back up my theory, but there was simply no other explanation for kidney cancer in both of us at exactly the same time. So, we threw away the charcoal grill, bought a gas grill, and went on down the road.

Just before Christmas, we finished the year by solving one last medical mystery. After healing from kidney surgery, Gerry still had belly pain. He went back to the doctor, and an endoscopy revealed a tiny stone left over from when his gallbladder was removed. The doctor sucked out the stone and sent him home. Problem solved. Pain gone.

That insignificant gallstone was another miracle in our lives. The pain caused by the stone prompted Gerry to go to the doctor. If the stone had not been there, it's doubtful doctors would have found his kidney cancer in time. The cancer was already stage 3. If not for the gallstone, the cancer could easily have reached his lymph nodes and spread throughout his body. God was clearly at work in our lives.

Joy and gratitude filled our home that Christmas. We were happy to see the year end, which we now jokingly referred to as "the year of the scar." We thanked God for giving us the strength to endure and rejoiced in the fact we had survived enough medical drama to last a lifetime. From now on, our lives would be nothing but smooth sailing.

CHAPTER TEN:
WAITING TO DIE, WAITING TO LIVE

Whatever is true, whatever is noble, whatever is right, whatever is pure, whatever is lovely, whatever is admirable—if anything is excellent or praiseworthy—think about such things. (Philippians 4:8)

Gerry and I coasted along for a few years without medical drama ruling our lives. Gerry's left kidney remained healthy. He felt great and stayed busy with his engineering company. For me, good health was a relative term. My heart was still too big. It still flipped out every so often and beat too fast or too slow or with an uncomfortable rhythm. But it kept on chugging, beating strongly enough to keep me alive.

Jeremy and Colleen welcomed their first child, a girl they named Laura, and Gerry and I drove to St. Louis to meet our new granddaughter. When I held Laura for the first time, all the years of fighting heart disease melted away. In that perfect moment, as I watched Jeremy care for his family, I closed my eyes and offered a silent prayer. *Thank you, God, for keeping me alive for this.*

The following year, Jeremy and Colleen completed their educations and the family moved to Dallas where Jeremy set up his practice as a licensed professional counselor and Colleen began her career as a pediatrician. It was great to have them back in the Lone Star State, where all four of our adult children now lived. Dana had settled in Fort Worth with her husband Josh and two children, Alyx and Aidan. Jonathan and Darren both lived in Houston. Gerry and I were delighted. Not only were our children physically close to us, they were close to each other and could laugh together in the good times and support each other through the challenging times.

Heart disease was a tenacious scoundrel, always lurking in the background, waiting to reveal itself and disrupt my life. Gradually, the physical demands of my job as a middle school language arts teacher became a struggle. I kept bottles of water on my desk because when I talked for more than a few minutes, I coughed and couldn't catch my breath. Walking across the classroom became a challenge, and lugging armfuls of books to school and back impossible. I could no longer give my students the one hundred percent focus they deserved, so I made the difficult decision to retire. It wasn't easy for me. I had to admit out loud I wasn't strong enough to do my job.

After I stopped teaching, my heart perked up a bit with a more sedentary lifestyle. I focused on writing and landed a few more book contracts. I kept a low profile and immersed myself in research, reading, and writing. I visited with family and friends as often as possible, and to get a bit of exercise, I attended line dance classes at a community center near our home. But instead of the challenging advanced class I used to enjoy, I switched to the much more sedate beginner class.

In spite of my efforts to hold heart disease at bay, my symptoms returned with a vengeance. Weight piled on regardless of what I did or did not eat. Puffiness and shortness of breath returned. When I had to sit down in the middle of a simple line dance because I couldn't catch my breath, I took what I hoped would be a short break and stopped attending class altogether. Coughing kept me up at night, and I felt exhausted all the time.

Once again, Dr. Strickman prescribed diuretics to get rid of the excess water and asked me to monitor my weight daily. It continued to rise. He doubled the prescription dosage, then tripled it. I continued to gain weight, my energy disappeared, and I couldn't do anything without feeling worn out. All I wanted to do was rest. It felt like my body was out of gas and puttering to a stop on a deserted country road.

Dr. Strickman ran tests in his office. When he walked into the examination room after analyzing the results, the sober expression on his face told us the news was not good.

"You need to be in the hospital," he said.

Not the news I was hoping to hear.

"Can we try some super strong medicine and let me go home instead?"

"No," said Dr. Strickman. "I've already called the hospital and told them you're on your way."

"Okay," said Gerry. "I'll take her right now."

"That won't be necessary," said Dr. Strickman, "a nurse will be here in a minute with a wheelchair."

What's the big rush, Doc?

I gritted my teeth. "What about the new valve? Wasn't it supposed to fix my heart? I thought we were done with hospitals."

Dr. Strickman explained that even though the valve was working properly, the left chamber of my heart, the left ventricle, was still stretched out and pumping poorly. Tests also revealed an abnormality in the electrical impulses controlling my heartbeat. That was something new.

So, we'd solved the valve problem and the leak. Now my pitiful excuse for a heart had a muscle problem and an electrical problem. Who knew there were so many things that could break in a heart?

Before I could ask more questions, a wheelchair arrived, and Dr. Strickman's nurse whisked me over the covered bridge connecting his office in St. Luke's medical tower to St. Luke's hospital.

I was not a happy camper. It seemed no matter how fast I ran I couldn't escape the malevolent predator stalking my life. Heart disease always caught up with me.

At the hospital nurses set up IVs and pumped heavy-duty drugs into my veins. The diuretics did their magic, and the extra water weight fell off in a matter of days. I felt much better and hounded Dr. Strickman to send me home.

"Not yet," he said. "I need to run a few more tests."

"But I'm better. I'm good to go."

Gerry took my hand and squeezed gently. "Patience, honey. Let him do his job."

The tests finally ended and provided the information Dr. Strickman needed to plan the next step on my journey to heart health.

"You need a defibrillator," he told me.

Once again, I added a new word to my vocabulary, a word I had no desire to learn.

An Implantable Cardioverter Defibrillator (ICD) is a battery-powered device doctors place under the skin, just below the left collarbone. Thin wires connect the ICD to the heart. The device would monitor my heartbeat and deliver an electric shock if it detected an abnormality.

It sounded pretty dramatic to me. I didn't want a second mechanical device implanted in my body to keep my heart beating. So of course, I grilled Dr. Strickman to make sure the procedure was *absolutely* necessary. Without blinking an eye, he assured me it was. My heart was failing, and this would keep me alive.

Compared to open heart surgery, implanting a defibrillator was a piece of cake. Doctors used a local anesthetic, it was quick, and I didn't feel a thing. I left the hospital the next day.

Getting used to the new machine in my body was a bit trickier. I'm not a large person and the defibrillator felt huge in my chest. It stuck out and felt like a boulder under my skin. I like to sleep on my stomach, but that was out of the question. It was like sleeping on a rock. The defibrillator came with a machine, placed beside the bed, to monitor my heart during the night. Lights from the machine made sleep a challenge because they often changed color or flashed. I'd stare at the lights and wonder what they meant. Was my heart flipping out? Was this it?

Questions without answers raced through my mind. What happens if my heart gets really, really bad and without the machine, I'd die? Will the defibrillator zap me over and over again and keep me alive forever? Will it zap me if I go back to dance class? Push a cart at the grocery store? Pick up my granddaughter? Does the zapping hurt?

These questions and a thousand others invaded my brain at night and made me feel like a sleep-deprived zombie during the day. I tried to pray, but my mind wandered. I tried to read the Bible but found little peace in God's word. Even though I felt far from God, he continued to watch over me. My heart kept beating, and the defibrillator stayed silent.

I resumed my normal activities, determined to ignore the machine sticking out of my chest.

As a new year began and life's natural rhythms settled into place, I realized I was taking God for granted. My single-minded focus on replacing "heart disease life" with "normal life" had drawn my focus away from him. Sure, I went to church on Sundays and attended Sunday school and small group Bible studies, but how much priority did I give God in my day-to-day life? How much did I read the Bible on my own? How much did I pray? Not much.

I realized my relationship with God had become lopsided and self-centered. A "call if you need me" casual association. I prayed for forgiveness and focused on deepening my connection with God. I carved out time with him each morning for prayer and Bible study. I became intentional about applying his word to my daily life. I looked for opportunities to serve him by serving others. And I grew more thankful. Thankful for all the second chances he'd given me.

God must have had a lot more to teach me because my heart flipped out again five months later. All the familiar symptoms returned: weight gain, shortness of breath, and tiredness. I told myself I could fix it on my own. I ate less to slow the weight gain, rested as much as possible, and ignored the puffy feet that no longer fit into my shoes. I was desperate to avoid another hospital stay.

In June, Gerry and I went to Dallas for a gender reveal party for Jeremy and Colleen's second child, due in early October. A large tribe of family and friends gathered in their backyard and watched Jeremy pull the plug on a long, colorful tube. Blue confetti streamed down on the happy guests and everyone cheered, "It's a boy!"

We had a blast congratulating the happy couple, playing with our granddaughter, Laura, and catching up with loved ones. Sometime during the festivities my sister Chris noticed my fat feet.

She pulled me aside and said, "Your feet look terrible. Doesn't that hurt?"

"Not too much. I'm used to it."

"Have you gone to the doctor?"

"Not recently."

"You need to go as soon as you get back to Houston. Promise me you'll call him as soon as you get home."

I knew she was right—faking good health is exhausting.

But I was worried. Dr. Strickman had already tried lots of different treatments, and my heart was still a mess. With a new aortic valve and a defibrillator already in place, it felt like he was running out of options.

And I was running out of time.

CHAPTER ELEVEN:
NOW WHAT?

*Do not fear, for I am with you; do not be dismayed, for I
am your God. I will strengthen you and help you.
(Isaiah 41:10)*

I called Dr. Strickman when we got back to Houston,
and we began another chorus of a familiar song. I curbed
my activities, took the medication he prescribed, monitored
my weight, and prayed. The diuretics, designed to pull
excess water off my body, started at 20 mg, but the dosage
rapidly increased to 40, and then 80, and still the water
remained. My kidneys were not happy.

Determined to fix my heart and save my kidneys, I
followed Dr. Strickman's instructions and tried not to let
health concerns invade the rest of my life. My publisher was
in the process of reviewing my latest book-in-progress and I
didn't want to start writing a new book until I'd completed
the final edits on the current book. So, to stay busy while I
waited for editorial feedback, I worked as an online writing
tutor.

My weight continued to rise, and each pound stole
another bit of my energy and stamina. By the end of June, I

was miserable. Dr. Strickman called one afternoon and told me to head to the hospital. I needed stronger medicine, and the only way to get it was through IVs. At that point, I was so worn out I didn't argue. I couldn't pretend anymore—something had to change. I felt like overboiled spaghetti, limp and worthless.

I checked into the hospital and was taken to a room in the cardiac wing. Tests began immediately. The results were so bad Dr. Strickman moved me to cardiac intensive care the next morning. Nurses wheeled in all kinds of machines and hooked me up. They placed IVs in both arms, each with multiple lines, and attached so many bags of medicine they had to haul in a bulky rack with multiple tiers to hang them all. Machines cluttered the tiny room and pumped, hissed, and clanked beside my bed. I lost twelve pounds of water weight the first day.

They're either going to fix me or kill me trying, I thought.

Dr. Strickman called in the troops. He ran the show and sent teams of doctors I'd never met to examine me. They ran tests and more tests, huddled outside my door, and discussed my options. The tests revealed my heart was in end-stage heart failure. My kidneys were in bad shape and my other organs were shutting down.

To stabilize my heart, doctors inserted an aortic balloon pump into the large artery in my neck. Attached to the tip of a thin flexible catheter or tube, a long balloon placed in the aorta inflated and deflated to help my heart pump blood through my body. The other end of the catheter was attached to a computer console that sat beside my bed and controlled the balloon inflation with each beat of my heart. The device helped my heart pump more blood with each contraction than my heart could do on its own.

The pump felt grotesque sticking out of my neck, and I knew by the expressions on Gerry, Jeremy, and Jonathan's faces that my faking-good-health days had come to a screeching halt. All three of them looked scared to death.

When the pack of doctors came to a consensus about what to do with my failing heart, Dr. Ziad Taimeh, a cardiologist who specializes in heart transplantation, delivered the news. Tall and thin, earnest and very serious, Dr. Taimeh carried himself with the ramrod straight posture of a soldier. He sat beside the bed and slowly and methodically shared my abysmal test results. Gerry and I listened in silence.

Then Dr. Taimeh laid out my options: undergo a heart transplant and maybe live—or go home, say goodbye to my loved ones, and die. Of course, he said it a lot more diplomatically, but that's the message we heard.

The words "heart transplant" first appeared as a treatment option for me when I was thirty-nine years old. I didn't believe them then, didn't take them seriously. This time was different. The rack of IVs and the machine sticking out of my neck proved I was in a lot worse shape now than the first time I'd heard those words. This time, I knew I was down to my last option. I could feel it.

"We'd like to begin testing to see if you're a candidate for transplantation," Dr. Taimeh said.

"I've already done that," I told him. "I've been on the list before. When Dr. Strickman put me on the list years ago, he told me I could be moved to a higher position if things got bad. Can you get my old test results, move me up higher on the list, and skip doing new tests?"

Dr. Taimeh shook his head. "The testing you had done before was too many years ago, and your name has dropped off the transplant list. You'll need to be evaluated again to see if you qualify."

I groaned silently, and the expression, "Ignorance is bliss," flashed across my brain. The first time I was evaluated for a heart transplant, I had no idea what the testing process entailed. *Sure, whatever, do what you have to do and send me home*, I'd thought. This time, I knew what Dr. Taimeh was asking and it sounded a whole lot scarier. Did I really want to endure the rigorous testing a second time?

Dr. Taimeh turned to Gerry. "You'll need to check with your insurance company to see if they will cover the cost of a transplant."

Gerry nodded and Dr. Taimeh continued his dissertation. "If all the tests check out and your application is approved by the transplant approval committee, you'll be placed on the national transplant list."

"How long will all that take?" I asked.

"We should be able to complete the testing in a week or so," Dr. Taimeh said. "The transplant committee meets every Tuesday morning. As soon as the testing is complete, we'll bring your file to the next transplant approval meeting."

"What happens after that? If I'm approved by the committee, then what?"

Dr. Taimeh shifted in his chair and leaned forward. "The committee will recommend where to place your name on the list. Patients at or near the top of the list receive the first hearts that become available. Those lower on the list wait longer."

He reminded us of the severe shortage of available hearts and cautioned that some patients wait months or even a year for a compatible heart. "You may have a long wait time because you have a rare blood type," he added.

"After I'm on the list, will I be able to go home and wait for a heart there?" I asked.

Dr. Taimeh shook his head. "No, you'll stay in the hospital. Your heart is not stable enough to wait at home."

Months in the hospital ... maybe a year ... I could not imagine anything worse.

Dr. Taimeh saw the dazed looks on our faces and told us we could discuss the details later, after I was approved and placed on the list. For now, I needed to decide whether I wanted to start the transplant evaluation process or not.

I searched Gerry's face for the answer and found the same shock and fear that had my heart pounding against my ribs like a battering ram. "Can I talk it over with my husband?" I asked.

Dr. Taimeh unfolded his long frame from the chair and nodded. "Of course," he said. "Don't take too long, though. We need to get started on the testing." Then he shook my hand, shook Gerry's hand, and slipped out of the room.

After the doctor left, Gerry and I had no words. For a long time, we stared at each other in silence.

Calm down. Don't panic. Breathe.

After we prayed for wisdom, Gerry and I began the long discussion that led to the big question—should I, or shouldn't I? I felt if I agreed to the testing, I was agreeing to the transplant. It was pointless to undergo all those tests if I wasn't willing to go through with the surgery.

"We need to talk to Dr. Strickman," I said.

"Absolutely," Gerry agreed.

"We don't know Dr. Taimeh," I continued. "Maybe Dr. Strickman can come up with a Plan B. After all, he's kept me alive for all these years."

"Yeah, we'll talk to him," said Gerry. "Maybe he knows of a new drug or a new type of treatment you can try."

There was so much to discuss, so many decisions to make. Gerry and I talked for hours. If Dr. Strickman agreed with the transplant plan, we needed to make sure our insurance would cover the cost. What if it didn't? Would the hospital kick me out? We needed to research the hospital and make sure it had a competent transplant surgical team, as neither Dr. Strickman nor Dr. Taimeh would perform the surgery. We needed to research heart transplant surgery to get some idea of what I'd be getting myself into and what was involved in the recovery.

We tried to be logical and discussed the pros and cons. But agreeing to let doctors take out my heart and replace it with a stranger's did not feel like a logical decision. It would require a huge leap of faith—in the doctors, the hospital, and God. We thought about the impact on our family. Of course, I wanted to live. My husband and children wanted me to live. But would they want me to agree to something as radical as a heart transplant? Did I want to put them through a trauma with such an uncertain outcome? I worried I'd feel worse after the surgery and become a burden to my loved ones. That was the last thing I wanted to do. I'd rather pull the IVs out now, go home, and save my husband and children years of angst.

My thoughts tumbled over themselves and crashed against my skull. The heart is an essential organ that keeps a body alive. It's also fundamental to what gives life meaning. It's central to our relationship with God and others. God tells us to love him with all our heart. I love my husband and children with all my heart. Although I knew intellectually those statements are meant figuratively and not literally, the image of a heart full of love is difficult to ignore when faced with the prospect of discarding that heart.

Emotionally, I struggled. Could I throw away the heart that had sustained and propelled me through my entire life—through the joy of falling in love and building a life with Gerry, the miracle births of our children, and the crushing sadness of my father's sudden death? Would a new heart change more than my body? Would I still be me?

Ideas swirled in an endless montage after the word "transplant" became part of my personal vocabulary. When I dozed at night, I'd wake every few hours with new questions for the doctors. I'd search the tray beside my bed for a scrap of paper or a napkin and write down words or phrases so I wouldn't forget to ask the doctors in the morning. At this decision-making stage I felt like the Tasmanian Devil, my mind whirling and ricocheting from one worry to the next.

When Dr. Strickman checked on me, Gerry and I discussed the transplant idea with him. In his typical calm, direct way, he agreed with the other doctors a transplant was my best option. We tried to pin him down on a timeline: how long would I live with a transplant versus how long without one. He wouldn't go there, but he did stress that in his opinion, a transplant was the best course of action for me.

Gerry went home and researched heart transplant centers in the United States. If this had to happen, was I at the best hospital? At the time of his research, there were other hospitals ranked higher in heart transplant positive outcomes than Houston's St. Luke's. So, should I have the transplant at one of the higher-ranked hospitals? Since we trusted Dr. Strickman completely and knew he always acted in my best interest, we talked this new worry over with him.

"Do you think we should transfer to another hospital, one closer to the top of the national rankings for heart transplants?" we asked him.

"No," said Dr. Strickman. "I think you should have the surgery at St. Luke's."

"Why?" Gerry asked.

"Because I'm here," Dr. Strickman replied.

He then went on to explain. The transplant surgeons at St. Luke's were top notch, as skilled as any in the world. In addition to that, at another hospital, I'd be just a name. But at St. Luke's, Dr. Strickman knew every aspect of my heart disease journey. He had made every medical decision about my heart from the day I learned the organ had a problem. He would oversee my care and take part in every medical decision. Nothing would happen without his approval.

That put an end to the discussion for Gerry and me. Dr. Strickman's expertise had kept me alive for twenty-six years. Every time I was admitted to the hospital, he'd plop down in a chair and treat me like I was his only patient. He answered questions and explained procedures in as much detail as I needed, and he had never given me bad advice. I trusted him without hesitation. We'd also seen how the other cardiologists at the hospital deferred to him. His experience healing hearts had made Dr. Strickman a legend in Houston. If he said I should stay at St. Luke's, I'd stay.

Because my heart was functioning so poorly, doctors urged me to start the evaluation process immediately. They felt time was not on my side. Gerry and I agreed to proceed with the testing. If doctors found a problem in some organ and rejected my application, the discussion would end. If everything checked out, and I was placed on the list, I was willing to risk death for the chance at a more abundant life.

CHAPTER TWELVE: TESTING

Surely God is my help; the Lord is the one who sustains me. (Psalm 54:4)

Transplant evaluation testing began immediately, and thorough is an understatement when describing the process. Transplantable hearts are in short supply, and doctors give them to patients with the highest chance for a return to good health. Before I could be placed on the list, doctors had to make sure all my other organs were in tip-top shape.

Blood tests were the priority.

Early one morning my nurse flipped on the lights with a cheery hello and dumped an armful of blood collection tubes on the bed. "I need to get some blood," she said.

I stared at the pile, wide-eyed. "You can't be serious. I won't have any blood left."

She smiled. "Don't worry, you have plenty of blood."

I turned my head away and listened to the whoosh-click as she filled each tube, popped it out, and snapped the next tube in place. In addition to testing the blood for disease lurking in my body, doctors used the samples to figure out the best possible chemical footprint for a donor heart.

Doctors ran tests on all my major organs, so throughout the day patient transporters appeared at my door and whisked me off to various corners of the hospital for testing. I burrowed down under the blankets and did my best to turn invisible as they rattled my bed down hallways and squeezed it into elevators. If the test results weren't clear or if one of the doctors wanted more information, they ran additional tests. Many tests proved challenging as I was still hooked up to the aortic balloon pump and lots of IVs.

In some of the tests, doctors injected stuff into the IVs and watched it light up the target organ. In others, I had to lie still on a hard surface for what seemed like hours while they ran scan after scan after scan. During each test, I prayed, *please, God, help me through this*. Whether it was a test or a scan or a blood draw, he always answered those prayers. I felt his presence, and because he was with me, I was able to stay calm, breathe, and stop myself from slipping out the back door of the hospital and calling off the whole thing.

At one point in the testing process, however, I broke down and had a garden of Gethsemane moment. It came after a horrible night of machines screeching, red alarms flashing, and doctors and nurses racing in for the rescue. *I don't want to do this anymore*, I thought. *It's too hard. I'm done.*

I was tired, so tired. Tired of hospitals. Tired of tests. Tired of people telling me I was on the brink of death. I wanted to go home. But God, in his infinite grace, used my family and the compassionate hospital staff to coax me off the ledge of despair.

The more they tested, the more nervous I became. Bodies have a lot of organs crammed inside them, and I worried doctors would find an obscure problem hidden in the deep recesses of my body waiting to announce itself. I worried they would find new cancer on my kidneys. It felt like I was taking the biggest final exam of my life, and if I failed, I died. One blood test designed to detect antibodies in the blood made me particularly nervous. If the number was too high, it meant my body would reject a donor heart and I would not be placed on the transplant list. End of discussion.

My number was zero. It was the first good news we'd heard in a while.

Testing seemed to go on forever. I was like the kid in the back seat of a car on family vacation. Instead of, "are we there yet?" my refrain became, "are we done yet?"

The Fourth of July fell on a Thursday that year, so by the third, all my doctors had taken off for much-needed family time. Testing stopped, and I didn't see any of my doctors until the following Monday. Of course, a holiday skeleton crew of doctors popped in from time to time to check on me, but basically, I coasted through the long weekend. With so much free time on my hands, it was the perfect time for a family huddle.

All four of our adult children came to the hospital from different parts of Houston, Dallas, and Fort Worth. Seeing them was like a burst of sunshine in the drab hospital room. After hugs and kisses, they wanted to know everything.

"We're all adults now, Mom," said my counselor son, Jeremy. "You don't need to hide things from us anymore. You don't need to protect us."

It was hard for me to share my fear and anxiety with my beloved children. I still wanted to shield them from anything scary or unpleasant. Yes, they were all capable adults, but I didn't want them to worry or be afraid because of me. So, we talked about the transplant and went over what we knew about the procedure and the recovery.

Even though they seemed a bit shell-shocked to learn I needed a new heart, I was thankful they had been able to enjoy happy, carefree childhoods without my health drama hovering on a dark horizon. And now that they were aware of my heart condition, I didn't want them looking over their shoulders waiting for heart disease to catch up with them. "None of my doctors think my heart condition is hereditary," I told them. "They don't know for sure how I got it, but they feel confident it's not something I passed along in my genes. You don't need to worry about cardiomyopathy."

It was important to me that my loved ones agreed with the idea of a heart transplant on philosophical and moral grounds. I wanted everyone united in case things didn't go well. We'd never talked about transplantation, and I needed to know how they felt about doctors putting someone else's heart in my body. We talked about quality of life—would mine change for the better or worse with a transplant? Would I be chained to a doctor's office forever? I'd lasted this long without a transplant, maybe I should keep on trucking and hope for the best. We talked about all of it, and we laughed, cried, and prayed together.

When visiting hours ended each day and my family left the hospital, they shared dinner together and hours of conversation. His children encouraged Gerry and lifted his spirits after weeks of worry about me.

It was a weekend lovefest. I felt their love for me and saw how they cared for and looked out for each other. We were transparent with each other and voiced our thoughts and feelings without reserve. They supported me in every way a person can be supported, and I had the chance to tell each of them how much I loved them. I also had the opportunity to share with them the unique ways each of my children makes a sometimes-ugly world beautiful.

Watching them, listening to them, I felt abundantly blessed. Four incredible human beings, and I had the privilege of calling them my children. Each of them is kind, compassionate, smart, confident, and accomplished. Seeing them all together in one tiny room was impressive. I felt a new confidence and peace wash over me. No matter what happened, my family would be okay. They would lean on and draw strength from each other. By the end of the weekend, we were all in agreement. When I was approved for a transplant, and they all believed I would be, I'd get a new heart, get healthy, and carry on for many years to come.

I accepted the fact that I did not cause cardiomyopathy. I would not cause the death of the donor. Life and death are in God's control, and receiving a heart would be a gift from him. If God wanted me on earth, I'd get a heart in time and the transplant would be successful. If he wanted me in heaven, it would fail.

I also acknowledged God expected me to do my part. I couldn't sit back and hope to be miraculously cured. If I wanted to live, I had to fight for life. I had to do the hard stuff. And I would. Because I wanted more time with my husband and children. I wanted to see my grandchildren grow and mature, meet Jeremy's new baby, fall in love with Jon's future wife. I wanted to live.

My husband and children brought me to another important realization. If I had a heart transplant, I'd still be me. The new heart would simply be an organ in my body. A mass of blood and tissue. A new and improved pump. It wouldn't change what makes me, me. It was difficult to wrap my head around the fact that someone would have to die for me to live. I worried about the donor family, their heartbreak, their loss, and how difficult it would be for them to agree to give a stranger their loved one's heart.

I decided the best way to honor their gift would be to take care of the new heart, stay healthy, and live a life worthy of the gift.

But before any of that could happen, I had to be approved and placed on the list.

CHAPTER THIRTEEN:
YES OR NO?

For I am the LORD your God who takes hold of your right hand and says to you, Do not fear; I will help you. (Isaiah 41:13)

After I mentally came to terms with the idea of a transplant, I worried I wouldn't be approved. Then I worried I would be approved. I'm not a fan of pain. I'd had open heart surgery, experienced the broken sternum and cracked ribs, and it hurt. A lot. I wasn't looking forward to the pain part of the process.

As Gerry came and went in cardiac ICU, he met families with loved ones in different stages of the transplant evaluation process. Always a talker, he got to know them and they shared the ups and downs of the process. We celebrated when someone was placed on the list and mourned when an application was rejected.

My doctors returned to the hospital after the Fourth of July holiday on Monday, July 8. They reviewed my test results and ordered more blood work and one last scan of my pancreas. This last-minute test made me nervous. Had something shown up on an earlier scan? Would this new test end any hope I had of getting a heart?

At St. Luke's Hospital, transplant review meetings take place on Tuesdays. All the doctors with transplant candidates attend the meeting and present the file on their patient. A team of doctors reviews each file and decides which patients are approved and which are rejected for some medical reason. Those approved are placed on the national organ transplant list. The transplant review team also recommends where to place the patient on the list based on the severity of their illness. Those closest to the top of the list are the sickest, the people who need organs quickly to survive. If approved, depending on where I was placed on the list, a heart could become available in days, weeks, or months.

While we waited to hear if I was approved for a transplant, the publisher for the book I was working on at the time sent me an email. She attached the cover design for the book and wanted my feedback. I loved the cover and sent back a few minor corrections for the jacket flap. Then I struggled with how to tell her I was in the hospital on life support waiting to find out if I'd get a new heart. How do you word an email like that?

The book, *Apollo 13: A Successful Failure,* was scheduled to be released the following March to coincide with the fiftieth anniversary of the Apollo 13 mission to the moon. The entire marketing campaign revolved around the spaceflight anniversary, so adhering to the publishing schedule and completing the book on time was crucial to its success.

I had been working on the book for nearly a year. My editor and I had completed several rounds of revisions, and my publishing house had been working on page layouts when I checked into the hospital. I knew at some point I'd need to review the page proofs, words and photos arranged as they would appear in the book, but I'd hoped to be fixed up and home by the time the proofs were ready for my review.

Unfortunately, that didn't happen. The page proofs were ready for my feedback, and I was sitting in a hospital bed hooked up to enough machines to cause a citywide blackout. I had no idea how I would pull it off, but I'd never missed a deadline on any of my sixteen books, and I wasn't about to start now.

I agonized over the wording of the email to my publisher and finally sent it. The editor-in-chief was completely wonderful and offered to do the page proof review at the publishing house. But I wanted to do it myself. Writing a book is a solitary endeavor, and I wanted to finish what I'd started. I had spent hours at NASA and studied all the flight journals, every word spoken between mission control in Houston and the Apollo 13 astronauts in space. I'd learned about every space mission before and after Apollo 13 and read tons of books and articles about the space race between the United States and the Soviet Union.

I'm meticulous when it comes to editing, and there are always errors to clean up at this stage of the publishing process. Some mistakes are small, like a missing comma or period, and I knew no one would search for errors with more dogged determination than me. My name was on the cover of the book.

My publisher and I agreed I would do the edits for as long as possible, and they would take over when my situation changed. Gerry was not a fan of that plan.

"The book is the least of your problems," he said. "Forget the edits and let the publisher handle things."

"You don't understand," I said. "It's *my* book. I've sweated over every word, and I want to finish it."

"It's not important," he said. "Focus on your health."

"It's important to me," I argued, "and it will take my mind off all the transplant drama. Look, I'm going to work on the edits whether you like it or not. It will go a lot faster if I can use the larger screen on that iPad you got with your new phone. Will you bring it to the hospital for me?"

"It's still in the box," Gerry said. "We don't even know how to set it up."

"Call Jonathan," I said. "He'll know."

He didn't like it one bit, but my darling husband brought the iPad to the hospital along with a blank notebook and pens and pencils, so I could take notes. Our son Jonny set up the device with my email account and showed me how to use the machine. My publisher emailed the first half of the book.

I had never used an iPad before and was unfamiliar with the device in general and the keyboard layout in particular. But I thought the benefit of being able to read a full page of text on one screen would override my unfamiliarity with the device and speed up the editing process. As I was connected to lots of IV lines in both arms and the balloon pump in my neck, editing proved more challenging than I anticipated. The iPad, an older model, felt like it weighed fifty pounds. I tried to prop the device on the bed and position myself so I didn't have to hold it, but it kept getting tangled in the IVs.

I struggled to concentrate as doctors and nurses barged into my room throughout the day and bugged me with annoying things like taking vital signs and hanging bags of medicine. I wanted to lock the door and steal a few hours alone to focus on the book. Of course, I knew I was being ridiculous. The doctors and nurses were working as hard as they could to keep me alive, and I truly appreciated every one of them. But I needed a short break from the whole dying-of-heart-disease thing. Just long enough to finish my book. *After all*, I thought, *it could be my last one.*

Editing was easier at night, after my nurse brought in my nightly prescriptions and the hospital settled down to sleep. I worked through the night and had almost completed the edits when I pressed the wrong key on the iPad and deleted the file.

I stared at the blank screen in stunned silence, my heart pounding in my chest. *Beat-beat ... beat ... beat-beat-beat ... beat ... beat-beat-beat-beat-beat.*

No!

After several minutes, the shock of losing the file wore off, and I pulled myself together. Then I took a deep breath, opened my email account, downloaded the original file again, scrolled to the beginning of the book, and began typing the edits a second time. This time, I saved my work every few minutes so I'd have a partial document in the event of additional technical mishaps.

As night eased into dawn, it became more and more difficult for me to focus. Weary and brain dead, I pressed the wrong key a second time and deleted the file *again*. Obviously, I needed a brain transplant as well as a heart transplant.

This time I lost it. I cried, felt sorry for myself, and cried some more. Then it dawned on me that since my brain was obviously not functioning, I'd better figure out how to recover deleted files before attempting the edits a third time. Google has answers for every question in the universe and file recovery instructions were no exception. I wrote down the recovery steps in my notebook, recovered the file, and tackled the edits again. This time, I started with a partially saved file and managed to finish the edits. I emailed them to my publisher and settled down for a much-needed nap.

On Tuesday, July 9, my doctors presented my file at a transplant review meeting.

All day Wednesday, Gerry and I waited for news—was I on the list or not?

"You already have a mechanical aortic valve and a defibrillator," said Gerry. "They have to put you on the list. Dr. Strickman said there was nothing left to try."

"Yeah, but if the kidney cancer came back or they found something wrong with my pancreas, they could tell us to forget the whole thing," I said.

The conversation fizzled from there.

Late that afternoon, Dr. Taimeh walked into my room and dropped into a chair beside Gerry.

"You are officially on the national heart transplant waiting list," he said.

I blew out a breath and felt a heavy weight slide off my shoulders. "What's my urgency status?"

Dr. Taimeh smiled for the first time since we'd met him. "You're Status 1."

"That's good, right?" I asked.

"It's the highest status there is."

CHAPTER FOURTEEN: LIFE ON PAUSE

Do not be anxious about anything, but in every situation, by prayer and petition, with thanksgiving, present your requests to God. And the peace of God, which transcends all understanding, will guard your hearts and your minds in Christ Jesus. (Philippians 4:6–7)

The wait began.

The United Network for Organ Sharing (UNOS) manages the national organ transplant system. UNOS divided the United States into eleven geographical regions. Texas and Oklahoma are Region 4. When a heart becomes available, donors are matched to recipients (patients) by region. The location of the donor is critical because donated hearts must be transplanted within four to six hours of extraction.

UNOS stores information about each patient on the transplant list in a huge database that includes the patient's medical urgency, blood type, height, weight, and hospital zip code. This information ensures that when a heart becomes available, the computerized network matches it to a candidate quickly and allows doctors to save as many patients as possible.

The wait time for a heart transplant varies from a few days to several months. Doctors cautioned my wait time could be longer for two reasons. First, my blood type, B negative, is found in only 2 percent of the population, and my donor heart blood type needed to be compatible with B negative blood. Also, the heart needed to fit in my chest cavity and I have a small frame. On the other hand, I was listed as Status 1 on the transplant list, so we hoped I would receive a heart quickly. That was both bad news and good news. Bad news because it meant my heart was in horrible shape, and I might not survive the surgery. Good news because it meant I probably wouldn't have to wait long to find out.

If I had questions before I was approved and placed on the transplant list, they were nothing compared to afterward. They slithered into my brain at night and waged war against the possibility of restful sleep. I wrote down lists of questions and discussed them with Gerry so we'd remember to ask my doctors. We wanted to make sure the doctors understood our wishes before I went into surgery. If something went wrong during or after surgery, and I was unable to answer for myself, I wanted to make decisions as easy as possible for my family and my doctors.

"What about the defibrillator?" I asked. "Are you going to remove it during the operation?"

One of the doctors shook his head. "No, we'll probably leave it in. We can always take it out later."

That didn't work for me. I hated that thing. It stuck out and made sleep impossible. I wanted it out. "Will the defibrillator be connected to my new heart?" I asked.

"I can't answer that now," he said. "We'll make that decision during surgery."

It was not what I wanted to hear.

After surgery, I wanted to be clear about how far the doctors could go to keep me alive, how much life support for how long. For example, I knew I'd be on a ventilator until my lungs could handle breathing on their own. Once doctors had taken it out, and I was breathing comfortably, I didn't want them to stick it back in if something went wrong. After the transplant, I wanted to know who would be in charge of my body? Me, my family, the doctors, or the transplant director?

Gerry and I created an advance medical directive. We hoped this legal document would reduce confusion and ease decision-making burdens in the event of a medical crisis during or after surgery.

Most of the doctors, especially Dr. Strickman, took as much time with us as we needed. They patiently answered our questions and updated us on any heart offers the transplant team had considered for me. Some of the surgeons intimidated me. They appeared in my room like apparitions and disappeared just as quickly. At times, I felt like a peon in their lofty presence, afraid to open my mouth to ask a question. Jonathan, my cool, calm, youngest son, was an expert at smoothly getting the answers I needed.

With so many ideas whirling through my mind, I couldn't remember the last time I'd slept. One night, one of the nurses took my blood pressure, and it was very low. She took it again, called in other nurses, and brought in different blood pressure machines. It stayed too low to ignore.

Nurses came into my room every twenty minutes and rechecked my blood pressure. The numbers didn't improve. Finally, after checking and rechecking for hours, they brought in the on-call cardiologist. "How are you feeling?" he asked.

By that time, I was so tired my eyelids hurt. All I wanted was a few hours of sleep without interruption.

"I haven't slept in a really long time," I told him. "If you could please ask the nurses to leave me alone and let me sleep, I promise my blood pressure will improve by morning." I heard myself pleading with the earnest doctor who was probably younger than my sons.

He was fantastic. I don't know what he said to the nurses, but no one interrupted me until the next morning. I slept soundly for several hours and woke up feeling like a new person. When the nurse checked my blood pressure in the morning, the numbers were closer to normal.

"Much better," she said and smiled for the first time since I'd met her. As she rolled up the blood pressure cuff, she added, "You worried me last night. I peeked into your room every thirty minutes to make sure you were still breathing."

"Sorry about that, but thanks for letting me sleep," I said, touched by yet another example of the tireless dedication of the doctors and nurses at St. Luke's Hospital.

As the long days passed waiting for a heart, God quieted my fears. I stopped asking questions and accepted the fact that a heart transplant was a giant leap of faith. There were no guarantees. Once they wheeled me into the operating room, I'd have no control. None. Instead of writing down questions, I prayed. The church prayed. Family and friends prayed. And God stilled the panic coursing through my cells and gave me strength to get through the seemingly endless hours. Did I want a heart transplant? Absolutely not. But for reasons I might never understand, it was something I had to face. God gave me calm, comfort, and a deeper level of patience as I surrendered my anxiety to him.

From my bed in ICU, I continued to work on edits for my *Apollo 13* manuscript and answered questions from my publisher. Dr. Taimeh stopped by each day and updated Gerry and me on the search for my new heart. On one of his visits, he shared his theory on my damaged heart.

"I believe your heart never developed properly in the womb and was spongy at birth," he said.

I looked at Gerry. "We've never heard that before."

Dr. Taimeh continued. "As you aged, your heart deteriorated and stretched as it struggled to pump blood through your body."

"Is there anything I could have done to prevent it from getting worse?"

He shook his head. "Not a thing. Since your heart was damaged at birth, it was inevitable. Your heart was a ticking time bomb waiting to explode."

It was a relief to know I hadn't caused my heart problems, but it did make me wonder. "I was born thirteen months after my sister, and my mother smoked heavily throughout her pregnancies," I told Dr. Taimeh. "Do you think either of those factors played a role?"

"Possibly," he said.

The wait for a compatible heart felt like an emotional roller coaster. Every time Dr. Taimeh walked into the room we tensed. *Is this it? Do I have a new heart?* Some hearts that matched my blood type were too big. They wouldn't fit in my chest. Some were too far away. They wouldn't get here in time for a successful surgery. And others were turned down because doctors didn't think the heart was the best possible chemical match for my body. When Dr. Taimeh turned down a heart for me, it was offered to the next person on the transplant list. I prayed each heart found a perfect host and the person who received it would live a long, healthy life.

Days passed slowly. It was a strange, surreal situation—waiting for someone to die so I could live. I couldn't pray for a compatible heart because that meant I was praying for someone to die. I had to remind myself God chooses when we are born and when we die, not me. Even though I knew I would have nothing to do with my donor's death, I had to repeat that truth over and over again. So, I prayed for strength to endure the challenges ahead and for peace and comfort for the unknown family whose life would soon be shattered with grief.

My church family had been praying for me and Gerry throughout our heart transplant journey. Lisa, the pastor's wife, was praying for us one morning and felt a strong urge to hold a church-wide twenty-four-hour prayer and fast day for my transplant. She talked it over with her husband, and he agreed it was a good idea.

"I'll discuss it with the elders of the church and put something together for later this week," he said.

Lisa shook her head. "No. It has to happen today."

She created an email flyer and sent it to the members of the church. The flyer, *My Heart, For Her Heart*, asked the entire church body to fast and pray for twenty-four hours, from ten o'clock Wednesday night until ten o'clock Thursday night. It was totally optional, of course, a request not a command, to pray I'd get the perfect heart.

On Wednesday, I had been on the transplant list for one week.

That afternoon, Dr. Taimeh and a whole herd of doctors burst into my room. I knew right away something was up. They sizzled with energy, and Dr. Taimeh had a huge grin on his face. He spoke first.

"We have a heart."

CHAPTER FIFTEEN:
LONG NIGHTS, SLOW DAYS

Be strong in the Lord and in his mighty power.
(Ephesians 6:10)

Things got crazy after that.

In the previous week, Dr. Taimeh and his team had turned down eleven hearts they did not believe were right for my body. They explained why they thought this one was a good match. They shared medical information about the donor but gave no hint as to his or her identity. They were still running tests, but all indications pointed to this heart being a good candidate for me.

There was one small problem with the heart, however. "The donor had an infection and the infection could be passed on to you," Dr. Taimeh said.

"That doesn't sound good," I said.

"We'll give you antibiotics after the transplant."

"Maybe I should wait for another heart, one that doesn't have an infection."

"If you decline this heart, with your blood type, it could be a long wait for another opportunity," Dr. Taimeh said.

The doctors left so Gerry and I could discuss the offer privately.

"Why is everything so hard?" I asked. "Why couldn't he have said, 'We've found the best heart in the history of hearts?'"

Gerry took a deep breath and blew it out slowly. "Dr. Taimeh thinks you should take it. He said the infection can be treated."

I nodded. "Yeah, all of my doctors think I should take it, even Dr. Strickman."

Gerry looked at the blinking lights on the machines crowding my tiny room. "I think you should take the heart," he said. "We may not get another shot at this."

The transplant coordinator brought in the consent form, a doozy of a document, pages and pages long. Reading all the things that could go wrong did not bolster my mental health, so I skimmed the document and nodded as she went over the key points. Then I signed.

It was a long day. There are lots of logistical details to work out before a heart transplant. The process involves several teams of doctors, and the transplant coordinator has to make sure everyone is in sync. Dr. Strickman, my primary cardiologist, and Dr. Taimeh, my transplant cardiologist, played key roles and met with us several times throughout the day. The surgical team, headed by Dr. Alexis Shafii, and the procurement team, headed by Dr. Aladdein Mattar, also met with us.

Dr. Mattar stopped by my room for one last chat before he headed out to retrieve my new heart. He is a warm teddy bear of a man and filled the room with a calm confidence that gave me courage. Gerry and I were subdued. I thought about the person whose heart would soon be in my body and prayed for his or her family.

A nurse came for me at seven o'clock in the evening. Gerry walked beside my bed as she wheeled me to the operating room. He could go no further than the surgical waiting room, and as we kissed goodbye, both of us wondered if this was our last moment together. I thought of my children and grandchildren and wished I could hug them one more time.

Surgery began at eight. At ten, my church family began their prayer and fast vigil. Jonathan came to the hospital and sat with Gerry. They didn't talk much—they were too scared. They just sat together and watched the agonizingly slow hands of the clock. At four o'clock in the morning the head surgical nurse came to the waiting room and told them the surgery had gone well. I would soon be moved to recovery and then to a room in cardiac intensive care.

Gerry asked the one question he knew I'd ask when I could. "Did they take out the defibrillator?"

The nurse smiled. "Yes, the defibrillator was removed. Now go home and get some sleep."

I don't remember anything about the three days after surgery. From what I've learned from Gerry and the doctors, they were precarious days. My new heart started out somewhat sluggish and took a while to perk up. Doctors adjusted the antirejection medications and worked to find the right balance for the bags and bags of drugs dripping into my veins. Nurses took lots of blood tests and doctors monitored the results closely. Each day, the numbers improved.

When I finally woke up, I knew I was in a hospital, but that was it. Totally confused, I tried to talk to Gerry, but the ventilator in my throat made speech impossible. Desperate to communicate, I motioned like I was writing. One of the nurses found a piece of paper nearby and handed it to

Gerry. He folded the typed paper in half so I could write on the back and handed me a pen. My shaky handwriting was nearly illegible, but I scratched out a few questions.

"Why am I here? Where is Dr. Strickman? Does he know I'm here? Where is Dr. Taimeh?"

I had no clue about the transplant, and I'm sure Gerry thought I'd lost my mind. But he patiently explained I was recovering from a successful surgery, and yes, all my doctors knew I was here.

Not being able to communicate, not being able to connect with another human being was painful for me. I felt completely alone even though Gerry was by my side and nurses bustled in and out every few minutes. I was an island and no one could reach me. The fog in my brain ebbed and flowed. It eventually cleared enough for me to see I was not alone in the darkness. God was with me, and I could still pray. When I stopped fighting, stopped trying to control my circumstances, God, through prayer, banished the raging lion of fear stalking my mind.

On Saturday, doctors removed the balloon pump from the artery in my neck. During the procedure, the artery tore and a blood clot broke off and traveled to my brain. Doctors performed emergency surgery to repair the torn artery and placed a stent in the artery to keep blood flowing to my brain. Then they removed the ventilator.

When Gerry saw me after I returned to intensive care, he knew something had gone wrong. My pupils were huge and I seemed more out of it than I had been before the procedure. Doctors ran a CT scan on my brain and confirmed I'd suffered a stroke during the removal of the balloon pump. They ordered blood thinners and told us the clot would dissolve in a few days or weeks.

The stroke caused a raging headache and damaged a small area of my brain. I could speak clearly, but I had trouble remembering certain words. Forget about names, many were gone. I made mental cheat sheets to help me remember important names. For example, Gerry had recently hired two new employees, Hector and Oscar, for his engineering company. After the stroke, I kept mixing up their names. So, to compensate, whenever we talked about work, I performed a quick mental calisthenic: H for Hector comes before O for Oscar in the alphabet, so Hector was born before Oscar and is the older of the two. It was the only way I could keep from mixing them up.

Lost words presented a huge challenge for a person who makes her living arranging words. I need words! New worries replaced my presurgical angst. Would my brain get better? Would I be able to read? To write well enough to express coherent thoughts? How long would I struggle to find the words I needed?

There are no guarantees in a hospital bed, and my doctors were doing everything they could to facilitate my full recovery. I thought about what I could do to help the process along and decided to work on fixing my damaged brain. *Reading is a good brain activity*, I thought. *Maybe if I read a bunch of books, my brain will forge new pathways in the damaged section and fix what is broken.*

I emailed my writing buddies for book suggestions. Gerry picked up one of the books and took it to the hospital the next day. It became the first of many books I read in a quest to repair my brain and restore vocabulary and recall.

Reading was harder than I expected. When I tried to read, I couldn't focus my eyes to travel along a horizontal line of print. My eyes drifted down the page and to the right. My doctors assured me that was normal after a stroke and it would get better. So, I pushed myself to read that book. Unfortunately, the book we randomly chose was not an author I was familiar with. Instead of short declarative sentences, the author wrote long, long, sentences, sometimes separated by punctuation, sometimes not. Some sentences took up half a page. By the time I got to the end of a sentence, I couldn't remember what the beginning was about, and I'd have to read it again.

I enjoy books—love them, actually—but I didn't love that one. The plot was okay, the characters likable enough. But reading had changed from relaxation to hard work. I forced myself to keep at it and thought of it as brain therapy. I knew if I could finish that book, I'd pass a huge milestone on my road to recovery. So, I struggled through the book, page by painstaking page. Sometimes I had to reread a section multiple times to understand the author's intent. But I plodded along, and eventually, it got easier to focus my eyes to move horizontally across a line of print. It took a long time for me to finish that book, but when I did, I felt like I could conquer anything recovery threw at me.

St. Luke's Hospital has three stages of heart transplant recovery: ICU, for the days or weeks after surgery, CCU, the organ transplant intensive care unit, and a regular room in the cardiac wing. Moving from one stage to the next is considered huge progress.

After five days in ICU, I moved into a room in CCU. Phase two of transplant recovery came with a set of milestones I needed to reach before I could move into the final phase and then head home. I needed physical therapy to exercise my new heart and strengthen muscles that had been dormant for weeks. Doctors also wanted me to gain weight as I had dropped to eighty-eight pounds since I'd been in the hospital. Doctors constantly tweaked my medications and worked to find the right balance to keep my heart happy without damaging my other organs. A pack of doctors visited each morning and monitored my progress. They took lots of blood tests and ran scans of my heart each day. They also scanned my brain to monitor the aftereffects of the stroke.

Physical therapy meant walking the CCU hallways. It sounded easy enough, but it was actually an epic production. I still had tons of IVs, and four drains were sewn into my body beneath my sternum. Each drain pulled gunk from the area around my heart and dumped it into one of four large plastic containers. When it was time to walk, two physical therapists had to unplug the IV pole and the four drain containers and attach them all to a rolling pole. One of the physical therapists pushed the pole as I walked around the hospital wing.

My body was weak and wimpy, and I moved like I was 120 years old. The CCU hallways were crowded with equipment and groups of doctors discussing patients. We had to maneuver around this obstacle course with care so we didn't rip out one of the drains or IVs in the process. At first, one of the physical therapists pushed a wheelchair behind me in case I felt dizzy or lost my balance. Thankfully, I never needed it. The first day, I could only make one loop of the floor, but gradually, my balance and strength returned. Each day, I pushed myself to add another lap.

In addition to reading and walking, I tried to gain weight. A nutritionist stopped by my room, and we discussed what I could eat on a low sodium, heart-healthy diet that would allow me to put on a few pounds. Lots of high-calorie foods also contain tons of salt. I had to stay away from salt to keep my kidneys happy. Hospital food is not the tastiest in the world, especially the low-salt variety. After days and days of the same choices, I learned to stick with salads and lots of ice cream and desserts.

One night a nurse walked into my room and told me I needed blood to replace the blood I'd lost during surgery. I was not thrilled with the idea, but since I was on a mission to get out of CCU and into a regular room, I swallowed my objections and nodded. She hung the bag of blood, told me to get some sleep, and left.

I woke up an hour later cold and wet. Confused, I lifted the blankets and saw blood everywhere. It was disgusting, the smell overpowering in the tiny room. YUCK!

I called the nurse and asked her to please, *please* remove the nasty mess.

"No, you need blood," she said. "I'll fix the leak."

She helped me clean up, reattached the bag of blood, and I stared at the ceiling the rest of the night.

Clearly, this would be a long recovery with lots of ups and downs.

CHAPTER SIXTEEN: RING THAT BELL

I can do all this through him who gives me strength.
(Philippians 4:13)

In the early days of recovery, I sometimes felt like the transplant had stripped me of every ounce of my humanity. I could not envision what my life would look like after a group of physicians, scientists, and chemists finished piecing me back together.

I controlled parts of my recovery, how much I ate, how much I exercised, and how much I read. But many things were out of my control. I could not remove the tubes, drains, and IVs connected to my body, and I would not be able to go home until all of them were gone. I really wanted to get rid of the chest drains. They were heavy, cumbersome, and if I moved the wrong way, the weight of the drains pulled against the stitches holding them in place.

One morning Dr. Shaffi, my transplant surgeon, told me to lower the head of the bed and lie flat on my back. He was going to pull out the first drain, the one farthest from my heart. Before he started, he called my nurse and told him to bring in the supplies he needed. But the nurse was on the phone relaying information about another patient to his doctor. Dr. Shaffi and his team had to wait for the nurse to appear with the supplies.

I thought about the long, grueling hours Dr. Shaffi works and how he seems to be in a hurry all the time, bustling from one room to another making life and death decisions that would crush the average person. He did not seem like the type of person who shrugged off delays easily, and I did not want to add to his frustration, so I lay perfectly still, a statue on the bed. I certainly didn't want to irritate the guy who was about to rip a tube out of my chest.

The nurse appeared a few minutes later with the supplies. I closed my eyes and held my breath. With a couple of quick snips, Dr. Shaffi cut the stitches around the drain and pulled it out. When I opened my eyes, I was shocked by the length of the plastic tube that had been inside my body. But he yanked it out so quickly, it barely hurt. Yay! One down, three to go, and another step closer to home.

My days in CCU settled into somewhat of a routine. The wake-up call came at four o'clock in the morning when an x-ray technician slid open the glass door, turned on the lights, and struggled to wheel a bulky x-ray machine into the room for my daily chest x-ray. Then the nurses took blood and vital signs. Throughout the morning, patient transporters whisked me away to various corners of the hospital for tests of one sort or another. And then there was physical therapy (PT).

A pair of physical therapists appeared like clockwork every morning as exercise was a crucial part of recovery. If I had tests scheduled, we tried to finish our daily walk before the tests. Tests always took precedence as doctors needed the results as quickly as possible so they could adjust my treatment plan. Sometimes we had to postpone PT until later in the day, but we always found time to walk.

Walking was something I could control in a place where my control was limited. I worked hard to increase the number of laps I could make around the wing. It felt good to stretch my legs and be vertical after so many horizontal days, and strength returned to my body bit by bit. Before the transplant I had been as flimsy as a shadow, my body fading away day by day. Now I was like a photograph coming to life in a developing tray. Each day the image grew stronger.

After each walk, my IVs, wires, drains, and tubes invariably ended up in a jumbled mess. My favorite nurse tried to find ways to keep them from getting tangled. When I got out of bed, he held some of them over my head and I ducked beneath. Or I turned clockwise, or counterclockwise, or stepped over some of the lines and under others. It didn't matter what kind of dance we tried. The lines looked like spaghetti all the time.

He spent hours in my room patiently untangling each IV line, labeling it, bundling certain lines together, and rehanging bags of medicine in an organized pattern on the IV rack. In fact, he did all his nursing chores with the same compassion and attention to detail. On one of my walks, I noticed a stack of cards and a colorful box attached to the wall in the hallway. Patients could use the cards to write commendations for any member of the hospital staff, and recognized nurses received extra compensation from the hospital. I wrote a card to express my thanks to the kind young nurse who went far beyond the call of duty to make my life easier, and Jonathan dropped it in the box. I don't know if the award committee was able to read my shaky handwriting or if my hero nurse received the award, but I hoped the hospital knew how lucky they were to have him.

Doctors and nurses monitored my weight daily and continually urged me to eat, eat, eat. They wanted me to gain weight before I left the hospital. I tried, but often when I thought I'd have time to order a meal, someone would come in and whisk me away for another test or procedure. Food services often delivered a meal while I was out of the room. After the test or physical therapy, when I had the opportunity to eat, I found I didn't have much of an appetite for the cold hospital food. In addition, my stomach had shrunk and I wasn't able to eat much of the food on my tray.

Food services delivered high-calorie protein drinks to my room several times a day, and I drank some of them. But it was impossible for me to finish all the drinks stacked on my bedside tray. I wasn't worried about my weight. I knew I'd gain all I needed and more when I got home. For now, I just needed to gain enough to convince my doctors I was strong enough to leave the hospital.

The longer I stayed in the hospital, the more I wanted to get out. The lack of privacy in CCU made me feel like my body was fair game to anyone who walked in the room. I endured the humiliation of being bathed by strangers as it was necessary to prevent infection, but I had to close my eyes and pray to get through it. I knew I'd have a lot more privacy in a regular hospital room, so I focused on what I could do to speed up my recovery and move out of CCU. My body craved sleep, but it seemed every time I dozed off, one of the machines beside my bed started beeping, or the patient next door started screaming, or one of the bags of medicine needed changing. *Okay, I'll sleep when I get home ... please, let me go home.*

One of the protocols for a heart transplant requires regular biopsies of the new heart to check for signs of rejection. My first biopsy took place on Thursday, one week after surgery. Using a local anesthetic, Dr. Taimeh numbed the area on my neck surrounding the jugular vein. Then he made a small incision and ran a long tube down the vein and into my heart. At the end of the tube small jaws snipped a piece of tissue from the heart. Dr. Taimeh and his assistant repeated the process until they had several samples of heart tissue.

I needed a new IV for the procedure, and that was a problem. My veins had been punctured so many times it was tricky to put in the IV. When the nurse couldn't find a vein, she tried another spot, and another. It wasn't fun.

The first time Dr. Taimeh snipped off a piece, my heart flipped out. It felt like it tried to jump out of my chest and then pounded erratically for several minutes. I was hooked up to lots of monitors and when the numbers went through the roof, Dr. Taimeh peeled back the sterile wrap covering my face and asked, "Are you okay?"

"Yes, I'm fine," I said, "but that felt really weird. Are we done?"

"Not yet," said Dr. Taimeh. "We need a few more samples."

I wasn't thrilled with the idea of repeating this procedure multiple times. A lot of people had gone to a lot of trouble to give me this beautiful new heart, and I wanted to protect it and let it get used to my body. *Leave the poor thing alone*, I thought. Then I reminded myself I am not a doctor, and I needed to trust the brilliant team that had given me new life. If biopsies were the best way to check for signs of rejection and get me out of the hospital, then bring on the biopsies.

The goal of a biopsy was to take samples from the apex of the right ventricle. This meant the tube had to travel through the jugular vein to the very bottom region of the heart. But because my new heart is a bit big for my chest, Dr. Shaffi had to angle its position during surgery for the best possible fit. Its position made getting good biopsy samples difficult because the thin tube bent as doctors tried to thread it down into the lower region of the right ventricle. Dr. Taimeh was not satisfied with the samples he was able to retrieve.

For the second biopsy a week later, Dr. Taimeh came armed with a new technique. He threaded a rigid tube through my jugular vein and then fed the biopsy instrument through the tube. In this way he was able to reach the lower area of the right ventricle and get the samples he needed. I had another biopsy the following week and then four more spaced out over several months. They all returned the same good news: mild rejection. My new heart was happy.

As much as I wanted to remove everything chaining me to the hospital, I was not looking forward to getting the stitches on my chest removed. There were a lot of stitches.

Dr. Shaffi, typically a man of few words, sat on the edge of my bed and talked more than I had ever heard him talk. All the while, he flicked his wrist and quick as a flash, pulled out stitch after stitch after stitch. When he was done, he smiled, also a rare treat, and moved on to his next patient.

"That was amazing," I told Gerry. "It didn't even hurt."

"Well, he is one of the best."

I smiled, closed my eyes, and said a quick thank you prayer. God was still with us, doing his thing.

To move out of intensive care and into a room on the cardiac wing, I had to pass a physical therapy test. My two PT walking buddies put me through a series of exercises:

walking, pushing against a wall, climbing stairs, and balancing from different positions. I passed everything with flying colors except one balance test. I got dizzy standing on one leg with my eyes closed.

"If you let me go home, I promise I won't stand on one leg with my eyes closed," I told them.

They signed my release.

On the last day of July, I reached a huge milestone—phase three of heart transplant recovery. Before I left intensive care and moved to a regular room, I had one last task to perform. Attached to the wall near the door leading out of the unit sits a large gold bell with a long chain attached to the clapper. The nurses on the unit lined the hallway to offer one last bit of encouragement. They clapped and cheered as I rang the bell three times to celebrate reaching the third phase of recovery.

I moved into a room in the cardiac wing on the twelfth floor. It was a larger room, and best of all, it had a window with a view of the sky and the promise of home. Recovery was a downhill coast from there. When physical therapy released me, they encouraged me to walk as much as possible on my own. I picked up the pace and walked around the much larger unit several times a day.

Gerry walked beside me, still worried I'd get dizzy and fall. "You've done enough for one day," he said. "Why don't you rest for a while?"

"Not yet. I can do another lap." And we circled the floor again.

Nurses removed IVs one by one, and one of the doctors pulled out the fourth chest drain. Dr. Mattar removed all the remaining stitches and talked with me for a long time about gaining weight. Incredibly kind and earnest, he encouraged me to eat, eat, and then eat some more.

"You need lots of protein," he said, "lots of steak and red meat."

I assured him I'd pile on the pounds when I got home, although he wasn't thrilled with my menu plan—spaghetti for meals and ice cream for snacks.

I left the hospital the first Monday in August. I'd been there six weeks.

As I stepped into the fresh air and climbed into the car for the ride home, a tidal wave of emotions washed over me. I will never be able to say thank you enough. To the dozens and dozens of dedicated doctors and nurses who worked tirelessly to give me back my life. To the donor family and the unknown person whose heart was now my heart. To my dear husband, my children, family, and friends for their unwavering support. To my church family for their countless prayers. To the scores of people who took the time to send an encouraging card or letter. So many debts I can never repay.

My eyes filled with tears and I thanked God, the one who controlled it all. I can never say thank you to him enough. But I would try to find his purpose in keeping me alive.

CHAPTER SEVENTEEN:
HOME AT LAST

For the Spirit God gave us does not make us timid, but gives us power, love, and self-discipline. (2 Timothy 1:7)

We pulled into our cul-de-sac, and the first thing I saw was a huge Welcome Home sign in the yard. Gerry was as surprised as I was. We found out later a dear friend had put it up while Gerry was at the hospital picking me up.

When I walked through the back door and stepped into my kitchen for the first time, it felt like being wrapped in a cozy blanket. I could sleep in my own comfy bed, eat what I wanted, take a shower, and use the restroom without someone hovering beside me. Things I once took for granted now seemed precious.

My first order of business was a shower. I wanted to wash my hair and scrub the hospital off my body. Taking a shower required being in a bathroom, and our bathroom contained a large mirror over the sinks. When I saw myself for the first time, I was shocked and horrified. My face was fat and puffy from the steroids I was taking to prevent organ rejection. It looked like I'd been blown up with a bicycle pump. I'd lost so much weight my skin hung off my bones like a concentration camp survivor. Then there were the scars. The big one, of course, from my neck down the center of my chest, but also scars from the defibrillator, the biopsies, the four drains, and the IV lines, on my arms, my legs, and my neck. My whole body was one red, angry-looking scar.

My weak and puny arms felt like they weighed four tons each, so the simple act of washing my hair felt like an Olympic event. After the shower, I brushed my hair and came away with handfuls of hair. It was falling out big time.

So, my future as a transplant survivor will be in a skinny, scarred, bald body?

I was back home, but I was by no means back to normal. It hit me with the force of a Mack truck that coming home was merely the first step on a long road to recovery. The doctors, nurses, and St. Luke's Hospital had done their part. The rest was up to me, and in that first shower, I caught a glimpse of the rugged terrain of the journey ahead.

A memory from my first day of teaching, right out of college, whooshed across my brain. All the new teachers had to attend workshops the week before classes started, and some of them were "getting to know you" activities. I was paired with another new teacher, and we had to sit on the floor across from each other and stare at each other in silence for three minutes. At the end of that time, we had to tell each other what we saw. It was meant to heighten our skills of perception.

When it was her turn to share, my partner looked at me for a long time, shrugged, and said, "I don't see anything."

It hurt my feelings at the time—was I so nondescript she couldn't come up with a single trait to share? But now, freshly home with my new heart, being invisible was exactly what I wanted to be. Not the sick person, not the heart transplant survivor. Invisible sounded perfect.

As part of my hospital release paperwork, my nurse gave me a notebook with important information about transplant recovery. I sat down, read the book from cover to cover, and hoped I'd be able to retain the pages and pages of recommendations. Then I pulled out the binder the hospital had given me twenty years earlier to see how much had changed in the world of heart transplants. The original binder consisted of a set of typed pages bound together with plastic coil binding. The current version had glossy professionally typeset color pages and a whole lot more information about how to thrive after a transplant. I noticed new antirejection drugs and reflected on how many medical advances had taken place in the intervening years and how blessed I was to have been able to stall the transplant for twenty years.

My *New Heart* binder included charts to record my weight, blood pressure, heart rate, and temperature twice a day. Any sudden changes signaled trouble and required a call to my transplant team. I dutifully recorded the required information and created my own critical path for healing. I focused on completing tasks that aided my recovery and ignoring anything that didn't. There were no doctors or nurses around to tell me what to do. I had to set the pace and keep myself moving forward. It wasn't always easy. Sometimes I felt like a science experiment gone wrong.

There was good and bad in my situation, depending on what I looked for. I was still alive, but I felt like hammered cat food. My new heart was beating great, so I prayed and asked God to help me focus on the positives. I'd eat a lot, gain weight, exercise, and somehow find as much of the old me as I could within this shattered shell. I'd ask my hairdresser for tips to arrest hair loss. I doubted there were enough exercises in the world to bring back the muscle tone I'd had before surgery, but I'd work hard to fix what I could in my wreck of a body. *Focus on the miracle*, became my silent mantra.

Addiction to pain pills is a very real danger after any kind of major surgery. I didn't want to usher in a whole new set of problems, so I rationed myself to one pain pill at bedtime to help me sleep. When they ran out, that was it. I would not ask for a refill. During the day, I tried to stay busy and ignore the pain. Sometimes it was difficult. I'm not a doctor and I didn't know if what I was experiencing was regular post-transplant pain or rejection pain. I figured if it was rejection, my body would let me know sooner or later, so I tried to live in the moment and look for beauty and grace each day.

Gerry had collected all the cards and notes family and friends had sent while I was in the hospital. He stored them in a beautiful gift bag and set the bag in my office at home. I spent days curled up in a comfy chair and read each card and note of encouragement. Card stores must have done a banner business that summer because there were cards from family, cards from neighbors, cards from church friends, cards from writing friends, cards from teaching friends, cards from line dance friends, and cards from fellow volunteers in a women's prison ministry. Many cards contained Bible verses, and the Scriptures soothed my battered soul.

I don't know how all those people found out about my transplant, but somehow, the word spread and kindness poured in. After I read, reread, savored, and cried over the cards, I stored them in a special box to be read anytime I felt blue. Little by little, I organized my office, cleared the clutter that had accumulated during my time in the hospital, and hoped I'd feel like creating magic with words one day. The opportunity presented itself sooner than I expected. My publisher called and asked if I could write photo captions for my *Apollo 13* book-in-progress. Real work to do? You bet, absolutely, of course, YES! An excellent way to ease out of sick-person mode and take the first step back into the writing life.

Dr. Taimeh performed my third biopsy the Thursday after I got home. The procedure went fine, and the results were the same as the first two: mild rejection. My new heart was happy, but Dr. Taimeh was not. He was concerned about a potential new threat and ran scans to check things out.

"You have a blood clot in the vein in your groin," he said.

It wasn't a big surprise. I could feel the hard lump, and since doctors had passed tubes through the vein during surgery, and as I don't have the greatest veins in the world, the vein must have been damaged in the process. "Okay," I said. "Can you write a prescription for blood thinners to fix it?"

Dr. Taimeh frowned and shook his head. "There is a chance the clot will break loose and travel to your heart or brain. You need to be in the hospital."

We were standing in a hallway in the basement of the hospital outside the scan room. My knees buckled, and I slumped against the wall. *No, please, no. I can't go back in the hospital. I've only been home four days! No. Just no.*

I took a breath and reined in the urge to scream like a banshee. "Tomorrow is Friday," I said. "The hospital will be deserted over the weekend. I'll sit in a chair at home and take whatever medicine will fix the clot. I promise, I won't move."

But pleading and bargaining did not sway Dr. Taimeh. He looked at me calmly and said, "If the blood clot breaks off and travels to your heart or brain, you will die. You need to be in the hospital."

After surviving a heart transplant, it was a warning I couldn't ignore. I checked my grumpy self into the hospital and sat in my room all weekend. I took blood thinners to dissolve the clot and read a book. On Sunday evening, one of the doctors on Dr. Taimeh's team took pity on me and sent me home. Since no one could predict whether the blood clot would break off or dissolve, he thought it was pointless for me to wait around in the hospital for something that could take weeks or even months to resolve itself.

Gerry and I couldn't get out of that hospital fast enough. We didn't wait for a wheelchair, as hospital policy recommends. As soon as the release papers were signed, we tore out of there and didn't look back. Of course, I had to take blood thinners at home and monitor my INR levels, but since I'd done that for years, I didn't think it would be a problem.

It was. The first time I tried to use the INR machine at home, I couldn't remember how to work the machine. I'd heard brain fog sometimes happens after long surgeries and can take months to resolve, but I thought I'd dodged that bullet. No such luck. The INR machine had a computer chip that needed to be inserted a certain way to read the blood sample I took by pricking my finger. I could not figure out how to insert the chip, although I'd done the test hundreds of times through the years. I kept sticking my finger, getting new samples, and the stupid machine would not work.

To say I was frustrated is the understatement of the century. I felt like I'd lost my mind. Finally, after I ran out of fingers to abuse, I called the help desk number on the machine and a nurse walked me through the process. As she explained the procedure, something clicked in my brain, and I knew exactly what to do. After that, I was able to calm down enough to collect the samples without a problem.

The blood clot in my vein eventually dissolved, and I moved on to the next hurdle on the road to heart health.

CHAPTER EIGHTEEN: ONE STEP FORWARD, TWO STEPS BACK

He gives strength to the weary and increases the power of the weak. (Isaiah 40:29)

Heart transplant survivors take tons of prescriptions, and managing the medications was a major undertaking. The hospital provided a large pill container with slots for four times a day for seven days. Gerry sat with me at the dining room table and helped me fill the twenty-eight slots. The antirejection drugs were the most important, and the dosage on those changed as my blood tests and biopsy results changed. At first, I took five in the morning and six at night of one drug and three in the morning and three at night of the other. Some drugs I took once a day in the morning. Others, once a day at night. One drug I took three times a day. Another, three days a week. It seemed overwhelming. What if I did it wrong? Would I drop dead?

Doctors stressed the importance of taking the drugs at the same time every day. The antirejection medication needed to be taken every twelve hours to keep the level in my blood stable. As the weeks passed, it grew easier to adhere to the medication schedule, and filling the pill container became a routine household chore, as simple as washing clothes.

I thought it would be easy to gain weight, but putting on pounds became a dance with one step forward, two steps back. Like most women, issues with my weight had always centered around trying to lose it rather than gain it. Now I faced the opposite problem, and gaining weight turned out to be harder than it sounded. I was on a low-salt diet and my favorite foods, Italian and Mexican, are loaded with salt. I hadn't eaten much in six weeks, and my stomach had shrunk. In addition, the antirejection drugs tore up my digestive system. Whatever I put into my body came right back out. I experimented with food and kept track of what worked and what didn't work. I set goals for myself. Ninety pounds, ninety-five, and finally one hundred. I celebrated each milestone, and after I reached triple digits, relaxed my diligent pursuit of pounds.

I wrestled with body image shame. As I worked to gain weight, I reminded myself the number on the scale was not a measure of my self-worth. I ignored the media images that bombard women with subtle messages that we are not curvy enough or tall enough or athletic enough or pretty enough. After a heart transplant, my goal was to have a strong, healthy body. I refused to let the number on the scale define me. If I was a bit too thin—so what? If I grew chubby—who cares?

As my recovery focused heavily on food, I experimented with new recipes. Gerry is more of a food fan than I am, and after the millions of sweet things he had done for me during my journey to heart health, I wanted to make tasty, low-salt meals he would enjoy. But my lack of cooking skills once again asserted itself every time I walked into our kitchen. I searched for enticing recipes, bought the ingredients, had them delivered to my front door, carefully followed each step, crossed my fingers, and hoped the meal would turn out. After hours in the kitchen, I couldn't care less about eating my latest concoction, but Gerry enjoyed my cooking experiments, and I gained weight, so the whole cooking thing turned into a win-win.

After a few weeks at home, I grew impatient with the slow pace of recovery. I chafed at being stuck in the house and craved my family and friends. But antirejection medication suppresses the immune system, which meant my body was vulnerable to any kind of infection. The threat is greatest the first three months after transplant, so my doctors urged me to stay home and avoid contact with people for three months. At first, isolation felt good. I was weak, felt wimpy, and needed to get my strength back. Pain was also a factor as well as my need to be near a restroom.

As days turned into weeks, however, isolation became more difficult. Life felt narrow, and I wanted wide. I longed to expand my world like a kaleidoscope and add splashes of color and light. Depression crept in, sleep became a hazy memory, and I fought my own version of PTSD—Post Traumatic Surgery Disorder. I had to force myself out of bed each morning. What was the point? Trapped in my house all day, unable to see my loved ones or hang out with friends, I felt sorry for myself and wondered why I had agreed to the transplant. Why was I still alive?

I needed to shift my focus. Recovery was going well. The problem was my attitude, and it was up to me to change it. When I was in the hospital, I didn't have time to reflect on the profound miracle taking place before my eyes. I was focused on accomplishing whatever tasks the doctors ordered for the day, doing my part to heal. Now that the crisis had passed, the full impact of the experience washed over me in waves of wonder. I was part of a small group of heart transplant survivors, blessed beyond measure and given a second chance at life.

Instead of wallowing in self-pity, I began to see the months of isolation as an opportunity to focus on God and the miracle that had taken place in my life. I read the Bible each morning and thought about God's love. Verses I'd read dozens of times now provided deeper insights. "And we know that in all things God works for the good of those who love him, who have been called according to his purpose" (Romans 8:28). *All* things, including a heart transplant. I focused on recognizing the good, finding the purpose, and celebrating the miracle.

In addition to strengthening my spiritual life, I filled the long days with activities to aid my physical and mental recovery. I walked around our house and cul-de-sac to strengthen weak muscles. Still concerned about the stroke and my spotty memory, I read lots of novels and biographies, learned sudoku, worked puzzles, played computer games, and read some more. My focus had improved and my eyes could now travel along a line of print, but as I read weightier books with complex plots and a larger cast of characters, a new problem emerged.

I found I had trouble keeping the characters straight because I couldn't remember their names. I'd start a new chapter and wonder, *who is this guy*? I had to flip back to previous chapters and check to see if he was the head of the French Resistance, the son of the closet Fascist, or the hidden Jewish violin prodigy. When that happened, I created a cheat sheet with character names and brief descriptions and stuck it in the book so I could refer to it easily. With those cheat sheets, reading became fun again.

As I grew stronger, my attitude changed. I saw each day as a gift from God, ignored the aches and pains of recovery, and let joy bubble through my mind and body. I started writing again—thoughts and ideas mostly, and then insights God had shown me through my journey to life. My new heart brimmed with gratitude and tenderness. Seeing my children on FaceTime or hearing their voices on the phone were moments to savor. Movies I'd seen a dozen times now made me cry. I cherished the little things—my husband handing me a hot cup of coffee in the morning, a phone call from a friend, the sun on my face as I sat in my backyard. I focused on the glory in the ordinary moments of life.

My transplant team ordered physical therapy for me in September to exercise my heart and strengthen weak muscles. I looked forward to gaining some independence, and of course, I wanted to drive myself. Gerry worried my driving skills had deteriorated with lack of use and thought I needed a refresher course.

"You haven't driven in a long time," he said. "You need to practice before you take the car by yourself."

"That's ridiculous," I countered. "I'm a great driver."

"Yes, you are, but you haven't driven in a while, and you're still weak. Humor me and let me go with you on a practice run."

So, I drove around our neighborhood with Gerry in the passenger seat, and, although I didn't admit it, found it harder than I expected to turn the steering wheel with my dumb wimpy arms. But I passed Gerry's driving test and took a giant leap toward self-sufficiency.

Three days a week, I drove to a nearby clinic and hooked myself up to a heart monitor. Then I walked on a treadmill and worked out on an arm-strengthening machine. As a former dancer, I've always had strong legs and good balance. The treadmill exercised my new heart and helped build stamina. At first, I could only walk for twenty minutes at a slow pace. Gradually, I increased the pace to a brisk walk and nearly doubled the time.

The arm machine was the bigger challenge. Upper body strength has never been my strong suit, and after two open heart surgeries what little strength I had was gone. I watched the black hands on the large clock on the wall every minute I spent on that devil machine. But I did it, three days a week for three months. The doctors were right—physical therapy definitely made my body stronger. I felt ready to conquer the world.

When I finished physical therapy, the clinic staff gave me a red "I Survived Cardiac Rehab" T-shirt and helped me work out a schedule to continue exercising at home. Fortunately, Gerry had purchased a treadmill years before, so it was easy to make exercise my first priority of the day.

One day out of the blue, the family of my heart donor reached out to my transplant team and requested an update on how I was doing with their loved one's heart. The transplant coordinator contacted me and asked if I wanted to write a letter to my donor family.

The request terrified me. I wanted to express my gratitude but couldn't find words powerful enough to convey the depth of my feelings. "Thank you" seemed way too small. In fact, every word I tried seemed too small. I wanted to write something profound and ease their grief over the loss of their loved one, but of course, that was impossible. Someone they loved had died, and I was still alive.

I prayed about the letter, asked God to please, *please* give me the right words, and after days and days of rewrites, finally sent it. That was my only communication with my donor family, but they are never far from my thoughts. I will honor their gift every day for the rest of my life.

My after-transplant quarantine finally ended, and Gerry and I started attending church services again. Our church family gave us a hearty welcome, and I was able to thank my friends for the many prayers they had offered on our behalf. My name recall problem asserted itself with a vengeance, and since I couldn't consult a cheat sheet for friends I'd known for years, Gerry often had to remind me of names that were now a blank to me. Our bond as Christian brothers and sisters was as strong as ever, so I didn't fret too much over the lost names. I just smiled, hugged, and chatted away like old times. I hoped the names would return with time, but even if they didn't, our connection in Christ was not diminished by the missing spaces in my brain.

Gerry and I finished the year on a high note, excited about what the new year had to offer. I felt strong, healthy, and determined to enjoy each day to the max.

And then the world fell apart in 2020.

CHAPTER NINETEEN:
BLESSINGS AND CHALLENGES

Come near to God and he will come near to you.
(James 4:8)

Gerry and I felt on top of the world as we celebrated the start of 2020. His business was booming, and he was excited about a couple of interesting new projects his company landed. I felt great, returned to line dance and tap dance classes, enjoyed lunches with friends, and picked up some freelance editing work. I also worked as an online writing tutor. The job allowed me to choose how many or how few hours a week I worked and filled my days with purpose.

Our grandson Ray had been born the previous October and because of my quarantine after surgery, Gerry and I had not been able to go to Dallas to celebrate his birth. In January, Jeremy and Colleen asked if we could come to Dallas to take care of three-year-old Laura and baby Ray for a week. Gerry and I would care for the children during the day, and Colleen and Jeremy would be home each evening after work. We couldn't say yes fast enough. Of course, we wanted to spend time with our grandchildren! As an extra bonus, our older granddaughter, Alyx, was dancing in a show that weekend near Fort Worth and we'd be able to watch her performance.

On the drive to Dallas, I was 98 percent excited, 2 percent nervous. I felt strong and healthy, but in the back of my mind apprehension wormed its way through my confidence. What if I wasn't strong enough? What if my heart went into rejection? Could I physically handle a newborn and a toddler?

God blessed the week in more ways than I could have imagined. Laura was a sweet-natured child and Ray an easy baby. I was able to get down on the floor with Laura to build castles and play games. We went to the park, blew bubbles with our bubble wands, and took long walks. Everything we needed to do to care for those children, God provided the means for us to do it. My arms grew sore from holding Ray, but they didn't give out. He liked to be rocked, so I spent hours in the cozy rocking chair in his room singing softly while he slept in my arms. Holding a sleeping baby is as close to heaven as I've ever been, and the months of pain and isolation melted away. If I hadn't realized it before, I now knew without a doubt that, yes, 100 percent yes, the transplant was worth it.

For the rest of January and February, I worked on publicity for the March first release of my *Apollo 13* young adult book. I created a flyer announcing the book's release and sent it to all the space centers and museums in the United States. I trolled NASA's website each morning and posted Apollo 13 stories on Facebook, with links to the book on Amazon. The Texas Library Association (TLA) Annual Conference was scheduled for March in Houston, so I worked with my publisher to schedule book signings and writing workshops at the convention.

In early March, I fainted. When I woke up on the cold tile of the bathroom floor, it took a minute for me to get my bearings. I'd had no warning and couldn't figure out what in the world I was doing on the floor. My heart felt fine, nothing weird going on there, but my shoulder hurt like crazy. I picked myself up and shuffled into bed, hoping my shoulder would feel better after a short rest. It didn't.

A couple of days later, I went to a medical clinic near my home.

"You have a broken clavicle," said the clinic doctor. He stuck my x-ray on a film viewer, flipped on the light, and showed me the break.

"No wonder it hurts," I said. "What do you do for a broken collarbone?"

"There's not much we can do other than to keep it immobilized," the doctor said. His nurse pulled out a blue sling and showed me how to place my arm in the correct position in the sling.

"If it doesn't heal properly, you'll need to see an orthopedic surgeon," he said.

I nodded and then pressed the delete key in my brain. *Had enough surgery, thank you very much. Nope. Not happening. I'm done.*

The worst part about a broken clavicle was having my right arm in a sling. I'm completely right-handed, and not being able to use my right hand presented more than a few challenges. I moved my mouse to the left side of my computer keyboard and taught myself to use it with my left hand. It was slow going. That little arrow went everywhere but where it was supposed to go, but eventually, I learned to control the thing.

My transplant team wanted to figure out why I passed out. I'm not a drinker, so alcohol wasn't a factor, and I'd eaten, so I wasn't lightheaded from hunger. As far as I knew, my blood pressure and heart rate were fine. So, my doctors ran a bunch of heart tests. Then they attached a monitor to my chest and watched my heart for two weeks. I wore a battery pack in a pouch around my neck, and the monitor recorded my heartbeats and sent reports to my transplant team.

Everything with my heart checked out fine, so we chalked it up to a fluke aberration. I saw the incident as another blessing. If my head had been the first thing to hit the tile instead of my shoulder, the damage could have been far worse than a broken bone. Unfortunately, passing out became a new thing in my post-transplant world. I passed out at home again and broke my nose, at church while chatting with friends before the service, and at a banquet in front of a crowd of strangers. Even though I didn't break bones every time, if it was possible for a person to die of embarrassment, I would have been a goner for sure.

Then COVID-19 hit.

The virus spread rapidly, became a pandemic, and Houston shut down like everywhere else. My book on *Apollo 13* was released with a whimper not a shout. The TLA conference was canceled, and I was not able to participate in any of the typical, exciting book launch activities. There were no book signing events, no school classroom visits. I couldn't even share copies with my line dancing buddies or my church friends. The world was closed.

I had lost nearly a year of my life with the transplant, and now that I felt great for the first time in years, it was difficult for me to stay home and isolate. I had envisioned 2020 as the fun year, the year I would finally be able to enjoy life with gusto in a strong, healthy body. Depression stalked my spirit, but before it gained a foothold, I turned to God once again. He reminded me he is still in control—even during a pandemic.

At the end of June, Jeremy, Colleen, little Laura, and baby Ray came to Houston for a visit. We spread a soft blanket on the living room floor for Ray and arranged stuffed animals around the perimeter to watch the fun. Ray's baby giggles and Laura's three-year-old chatter filled the house with joy as we caught up with Jeremy and Colleen. We played a ton of games, read dozens of children's books, and took long walks in the summer sunshine. It was the perfect weekend.

The day after they left, Gerry felt sick. He had all the symptoms of COVID-19.

CHAPTER TWENTY:
GOD'S NOT DONE

The Lord is near to all who call on him, to all who call on him in truth. (Psalm 145:18)

Gerry tested positive for COVID-19, and since the virus is most contagious a few days before symptoms appear, Jeremy and his family had been exposed to the disease the entire time they were in our home. Gerry and I treasure every opportunity we have to spend time with our children and grandchildren and were devastated they had been exposed to a life-threatening virus while they were staying with us. The two-week waiting period to see if any of them developed COVID symptoms was excruciating. Thankfully, none of them got sick.

Gerry felt miserable for three weeks, but he did not need to be hospitalized. The medication I was on suppressed my immune system, so I was considered high-risk for catching the virus. Much to everyone's surprise, I did not get sick and was able to care for Gerry at home.

While treating his COVID, Gerry's doctors noticed spots on his lungs and referred him to other specialists for further testing. He ended up at MD Anderson Cancer Center, and after a biopsy and several scans, we spent an anxious couple of weeks waiting to find out if the spots indicated a serious health problem. His doctors diagnosed the spots as Follicular Lymphoma, a slow-growing cancer of the lymph nodes. As the cancer was small, no treatment was required at that time, but the MD Anderson cancer team scheduled Gerry for periodic follow-up testing to monitor the cancer to make sure it didn't grow large enough to present a problem. We recognized Gerry's bout with COVID as another blessing from God. Without it, we would not have known to keep an eye on the cancer.

I reached my one-year transplant anniversary in July, and my doctors scheduled a bunch of tests to mark this important milestone. Dr. Taimeh no longer worked at St. Luke's Hospital; he had transferred to a hospital in Ohio. Dr. Ajith Nair took over my treatment plan. Small and wiry, Dr. Nair looked like he ran marathons for breakfast. He believed the risks involved with heart biopsies after a transplant outweighed the benefits, so he scheduled several noninvasive tests to gather the same information a biopsy would have provided. I was totally on board with his plan.

The tests were stacked one after another from eight o'clock in the morning to four o'clock in the afternoon. I knew it would be a long day when the blood-draw nurse couldn't get blood from my right arm and had to stick me again on the left. Then the CT scan people had to put in an IV and pump drugs into my veins to slow my heart rate because my heart was beating too fast to get an accurate image on the scan. But the minor testing glitches didn't faze me. I felt terrific, and I knew my heart was happy in its new home. On the way home from the hospital, Gerry and I stopped to enjoy a delicious Italian meal to celebrate my first year of heart health.

The test results came in a few days later. My heart was pumping better than it had my entire life. No wonder I felt fabulous! A bone scan proved my bones were still brittle—no surprise there—and I'd have to do something about that, but every heart test returned positive results. Another miracle, far beyond our wildest expectations.

Some people thought I would change after a heart transplant. They thought my personality would change. They thought I would take on the characteristics of my donor. They thought my taste buds would change, and I would prefer different foods over my typical favorites. I have changed, but not in any of those ways.

I now see each day as a gift to unwrap as I step out of bed in the morning. I look forward to each fragile, precious, unpredictable moment. That doesn't mean I never get grumpy or angry or selfish. I still say things I shouldn't. I still struggle to trust God's plan for my life. I'm still a flawed human, and I still sin. But now I'm a flawed sinner with a strong heart. And my strong heart is a tender, thankful heart.

I'm thankful for everyday blessing—a hot cup of coffee in the morning, a text message from one of my children, being able to watch a wild rabbit nibble grass in my backyard. I treasure the simple joy of being alive and strive to honor the gift I've been given by living each day in a way that honors God.

I laugh more.

I cry more—at the sound of a loved one's voice, at movies I've seen a dozen times, at commercials, and at stories in the news.

I'm more patient. Things that used to frustrate me—Houston traffic, rude behavior, money woes, political insanity—I now see as no big deal. God is in control, and whatever it is will resolve itself, one way or another. Life is short, too short to waste it on arguments or petty squabbles.

I'm more aware and more intentional. Part of this new awareness stems from the fact I feel strong and healthy for the first time in years. But it's more than that. Every person on the planet suffers pain of one sort or another. We all face obstacles—disease, financial setbacks, job loss, shattered relationships, or the loss of a loved one.

My obstacles taught me two things. God is good—always. And if you trust him, he will use your obstacles to draw you closer to him.

Sometimes, I feel guilty for the gift I've been given. Why me? Thousands of people die of heart disease each year. Patients around the world wait in vain for transplants that never come. Others die in the operating room or shortly after surgery. Why does God allow some to live and some to die?

I can't answer that question. I'm not capable of understanding God's plans or of knowing the whys and why nots in every situation. I don't know why he allowed cardiomyopathy to invade my life and then blessed me with the perfect heart. But I trust him, and I know he used my heart transplant for my good, not just my physical good but my eternal good as well. It took a life-threatening illness to get my attention—I'm a stubborn sinner. But he loves me enough to create circumstances in my life to draw me to him.

I can never repay the gift I've been given. The price is beyond measure. What I can do is live each day in a way that honors God and look for opportunities to lift up others as countless angels lifted me. I can show sensitivity, kindness, and love to each person God puts in my path. I can share the message of God's love for us through his son, Jesus Christ.

You may never need a heart transplant. I hope you don't. I hope you enjoy perfect health. But whether you are fighting disease or in excellent health, at some point in your future, you will die. Investigate the claims of Jesus for yourself, before it's too late. Read the Bible. Find a church. Ask tough questions. Study. It's worth the effort now to ensure your future for eternity. This earthly life is short, and it will end. Eternity has no end.

So, this isn't my story after all. It's God's story. It's the story of his faithfulness, his love, and his awesome power. It's the story of how he led a selfish sinner on a journey and then called her to himself. I learned a lot about myself on that journey and even more about God.

May he grant you the courage, faith, and peace to embrace his plan for your journey.

PART II

CRIES OF A WOUNDED HEART

They will have no fear of bad news; their hearts are steadfast, trusting in the LORD. (Psalm 112:7)

God is good, yet suffering exists in the world. Can happiness exist amid suffering? I am not a theologian. I am not a preacher. I am a sinner who has suffered. During my seasons of adversity, I found strength in the examples of the biblical characters in the following pages. They showed me how to live well with suffering in light of God's word. I pray they will give you strength to face the suffering in your life.

Each of these men faced trials in his life, and each showed enormous perseverance. They did not abandon their faith in God despite their personal struggles. God does not promise a life of ease or monetary success. He does not promise a life of comfort. He does not promise to take away the obstacles in our lives. But Jesus does promise to be with us as we face our trials. He promises to give us the strength to endure them. And he promises rest and comfort for eternity.

JOB

I know that you can do all things; no purpose of yours can be thwarted. (Job 42:2)

Job was a man who had it all—good health, a large family, and great wealth. He was an honorable man, a loving husband and father, and he served God with all his heart. God called Job blameless.

Satan saw that Job was an upright man and wanted to prove to God he could turn Job against him. Satan believed the reason Job loved God was because God had blessed him with everything a person could desire. "But now stretch out your hand and strike everything he has, and he will surely curse you to your face," Satan challenged God (Job 1:11). God allowed Satan to bring suffering into Job's life. The only restriction God placed on Satan was he could not kill Job.

Satan wreaked havoc on Job's life. He took all Job's possessions, his livestock, and all ten of his children. Despite his losses, Job praised God, even as he grieved. Next, Satan sent Job a terrible, painful illness, and still, Job trusted God.

After a while, though, as Job suffered in excruciating pain, he began to question God. Why me? I am a good man, a faithful servant. How can you be so cruel to one of your own? Job began to doubt God's wisdom and fairness. He complained to his friends, and his friends told him he must have sinned, and God was punishing him for those sins. But Job knew he was a man of integrity who sincerely tried to please God. Job questioned God about the reason for suffering, and he cursed the day he was born, but he never lost his faith in God.

God listened to Job vent and complain, and he responded. Through a series of questions, God showed Job the vast chasm between God and man, the insignificance of man compared to God. He asked Job, where were you when I created the world? Did you create light and darkness? Can you make it rain or snow? Can you make a new constellation of stars in the heavens? Did you make the eagle fly or give the horse his strength?

Job could not answer any of God's questions, and he recognized his ignorance and impotence compared to God. He admitted his limitations and told God he had no idea how to control the universe. Job was not capable of understanding God's plan for him or how that plan fit into his plan for the world. Neither are we. Our human brains are nowhere near the mind of God, and as God showed Job, all our great knowledge and scientific advances are like a speck of dust compared to the power and wisdom of God.

In his pain, Job spoke as if he were wiser than God. But in the end, Job trusted God and was faithful. He asked for forgiveness, and God forgave him, blessed him, and gave him restored health, possessions, children, and a prosperous life. Job's story shows us we can bring our pain and grief to God and trust he hears us and cares about our suffering.

Job's story reminds me I am not in control of the universe. I don't know what God knows, and I don't know why he does what he does or allows what he allows. Job never finds out the reason for his suffering, and we may never find out the reason for ours. Many good people suffer. Many evil people enjoy success. Human wisdom attempts to explain this unexplainable dichotomy, but we cannot. Like Job, we are not able to understand every single thing in the universe. But God does. He planned it. He created it. He maintains it. God allows pain for his own reasons, but he may never reveal those reasons to us. He doesn't have to. He is God and we are his creations.

I can relate to Job. During my sister Chris's long battle with Crohn's disease, I questioned God, and thought I knew better than he did what was best for my sister. When he didn't heal her, I was angry and turned my back on him. I thought my prayers were evaporating in thin air, going nowhere, because if he heard them, surely, he would grant my request and heal my sister. I felt God had abandoned Chris and ignored my pleas for her.

Like Job, it took me a long time to admit God knows more than I do. He has a plan for my sister, and his plan is perfect.

Even when I don't understand it.

Even when I want a different plan.

Always.

SAUL/PAUL

We fix our eyes not on what is seen, but on what is unseen, since what is seen is temporary, but what is unseen is eternal. (2 Corinthians 4:18)

Saul was born a Jew. He studied under the top Jewish leaders of his time and became highly educated in the Jewish faith. He was also a Roman citizen, and as a young adult, he diligently worked to stop the spread of Christianity. Saul was so ardent in his persecution of Christians he went from house to house looking for Christians to throw in jail. He watched and gave his approval as a Christian named Stephen was stoned to death for preaching the gospel of salvation through Jesus Christ.

On a journey to Damascus, where Saul was on his way to hunt down Christians, a light from heaven flashed around him. Saul fell to the ground and heard a voice. "Saul, Saul, why do you persecute me" (Acts 9:4)?

Saul asked who was speaking, and the Lord replied, "I am Jesus, whom you are persecuting" (Acts 9:5).

After the light dimmed and the voice stopped speaking, Saul opened his eyes and stood, but he could not see. He was blind. His traveling companions led him to Damascus where he remained blind for three days and did not eat or drink anything. The Lord told Ananias, a Christian disciple, to go to Saul and restore his sight. Ananias placed his hands on Saul, his sight was restored, and he became a Christian. After he came to faith, Saul was called Paul.

Although Paul did not believe in Jesus in his early life and worked to silence others who did believe, after his conversion God used him in powerful ways to spread his message of love and hope. Paul immediately began to preach the message of salvation through Jesus Christ. He founded several churches, became one of the most influential missionaries of the early Christian church, and wrote half of the New Testament books of the Bible.

Paul's life did not get easier after he became a believer. In fact, instead of living a life of privilege and ease as a Roman citizen, his life became much, much more difficult. Paul faced many trials, and he suffered for his faith. He was attacked, arrested, accused of being a fake, imprisoned repeatedly, shipwrecked three times, beaten with rods, pelted with stones, flogged, and exposed to death many times. Paul also suffered from something he called "a thorn in my flesh" and described it as torment. Although we don't know what type of affliction the thorn represented, it is clear Paul suffered.

Evil things happen, and sometimes life is tragic. "I have great sorrow and unceasing anguish in my heart," Paul wrote (Romans 9:2). Yet Paul did not abandon God in his struggles. He did not stop working at the job God called him to do. He persevered in spite of the hardships he faced. Paul knew God loved him, and although he was sometimes discouraged, his life shows that pain, suffering, and sorrow can be endured through faith in Christ and hope in an eternity with him in heaven.

I can relate to Paul. For years, I turned my back on God. I thought the Old Testament of the Bible was a convoluted collection of stories that may or may not be true. I read the New Testament and learned about a good man named Jesus who may or may not have really lived. I had the head knowledge of God's plan of salvation for his people, but it did not penetrate the hard shell of my heart.

Paul's story reminds me God can save anyone. He can transform the heart of even the most wretched sinner. Even though I turned my back on him, like Paul, Jesus did not turn his back on me. He created circumstances in my life to draw me to himself, and he waited patiently to welcome me into his family.

When I get discouraged, Paul reminds me how blessed I am to be part of God's family. What happens to me here on earth pales in comparison to my future with Jesus in heaven for eternity.

An eternity where there will be no suffering.

SIMON PETER

With minds that are alert and fully sober, set your hope
on the grace to be brought to you when Jesus Christ is
revealed at his coming. (1 Peter 1:13)

Simon Peter was a Galilean fisherman. The work was
physically demanding, and Simon Peter was described as a
man's man. He was loud and boisterous, had an explosive
temper, and was impulsive. Simon Peter was the kind of
man who sometimes put his foot in his mouth and spoke
before he thought.

One day, Jesus was standing by the Sea of Galilee and
saw Simon Peter rolling up his nets after an unsuccessful
night of fishing. Jesus went into Simon's boat and asked
him to put out into deep water and cast out his nets
again. Simon protested. He told Jesus he and his brothers
had fished all night and hadn't caught a single fish. But
because Jesus asked, Simon once again threw out his nets.
He caught so many fish his nets began to break.

When Simon saw this, he fell at Jesus's knees and said,
"Go away from me, Lord; I am a sinful man" (Luke 5:8)!
Jesus reassured Simon and invited him to join him as one
of his disciples. He gave Simon the name Peter, which

means "rock," and Simon left his boat, traveled with Jesus, learned about the kingdom of God, and spread the gospel.

On one occasion, as Jesus was teaching a large crowd, a synagogue ruler named Jairus fell at his feet. Jairus pleaded with Jesus to come with him and heal his daughter who was dying. Jesus immediately set off with Jairus. On the way, a messenger arrived and told Jairus his daughter had already died.

Jesus told Jairus his daughter would be healed and continued walking. When they arrived at the synagogue ruler's home, they found a large crowd in front of the house, wailing in mourning for the dead child. Jesus took three of his disciples, Peter, James, and John, along with the child's parents, into the child's room. He took her by the hand and told her to get up. The little girl stood, and her parents gave her something to eat.

It is significant Peter was with Jesus in the child's room and witnessed the girl coming back to life. It shows the closeness and trust Jesus had in Peter and how Jesus was preparing Peter for his role as a leader after his death.

The night before he was crucified, Jesus and his disciples went to a place called the garden of Gethsemane. Jesus asked the men to keep watch while he went to pray. He took Peter, James, and John farther into the garden to pray and keep watch. Then Jesus retreated to an isolated spot by himself to pray. When Jesus returned, he found Peter, James, and John asleep. "Couldn't you men keep watch with me for one hour?" he asked Peter (Matthew 26:40). Peter loved Jesus and tried to stay awake and pray for him, but he was tired after a long day, and he fell asleep despite his best intentions.

Later that night, guards arrested Jesus and took him to Caiaphas, the high priest. Peter followed at a distance and lingered in the courtyard of the high priest so he could see what happened to Jesus. While Peter sat in the courtyard, a servant girl spotted him and accused him of being an associate of Jesus. Peter denied it. Two more bystanders accused Peter of being with Jesus, and both times, Peter denied knowing him.

Jesus knew Peter would reject him. He predicted it. "Truly I tell you," Jesus told Peter, "this very night, before the rooster crows, you will disown me three times" (Matthew 26:34). Just as Peter denied knowing Jesus for the third time, the rooster crowed. Peter glanced around and saw Jesus turn and look straight at him. He remembered Jesus predicted his denial and wept bitterly.

Peter loved Jesus with all his heart. He swore he would never leave him and promised he would even die for him. There is no doubt Peter was sincere. But Peter was human, and he had many flaws. Jesus knew Peter's shortcomings and loved him anyway. He did not abandon Peter or write him off as a lost cause when he made mistakes. Peter's story shows that everyone sins, even people with great faith, people who truly love God. But God does not abandon us in our sin.

Jesus had big plans for Peter. After he rose from the grave, Jesus talked with Peter, and Peter became an influential Christian leader. He changed from an uneducated, arrogant, volatile man to a humble, fearless servant of Christ and stayed that way until the day he died. Peter still made mistakes. He still sinned. Yet he preached the gospel boldly and helped spread the Christian faith to both Jews and gentiles.

I can relate to Peter. Like him, I have made mistakes. I have remained silent when I should have spoken boldly in faith. Jesus knew Peter would deny him at the time of his greatest need, and Jesus knows every one of our human failings. He knows we'll make mistakes and do things we're ashamed of later. Peter felt unworthy of God's love, and in his human weakness, he sinned. But God forgave him, loved him, and gave him the courage to accomplish great things.

Fear does not mean failure, and doubt does not mean death. Jesus knows our human frailty. He knows our fears and doubts, even the ones we keep hidden from the world and from ourselves. Jesus loved Peter and wanted a relationship with him, even though Peter sinned again and again.

He wants the same with us.

MOSES

Satisfy us in the morning with your unfailing love, that we may sing for joy and be glad all our days. (Psalm 90:14)

Moses was born a Hebrew slave in Egypt. Pharaoh, the Egyptian king, feared the number of Hebrew slaves being born and ordered every Jewish boy killed at birth. Moses's mother hid him for three months, but when she realized she couldn't hide him forever, she placed him in a papyrus basket coated with tar and sent him down the Nile River.

Pharoah's daughter found the basket among the reeds, took pity on the crying baby, and brought him into the palace. Moses's sister, Miriam, asked Pharoah's daughter if she could find a Hebrew woman to nurse the baby. Miriam brought Moses's mother, and she nursed the baby until he was weaned. Moses was raised at the palace as Pharoah's grandson and grew strong and healthy.

Moses lived a life of luxury at the palace. He was given the finest of everything, educated, and grew to be a man of power and strength. When Moses was approximately forty years old, he visited a worksite and saw how the Egyptians were oppressing and mistreating the Hebrew slaves. He killed one of the Egyptian foremen and hid his body in the sand. When Pharoah learned of the murder, he ordered Moses to be killed, but Moses fled from Pharoah and went to a place called Midian.

Moses settled in Midian, married, and had two sons. Forty years later, he was tending his father-in-law's flock when the Lord appeared to him in flames of fire from within a bush. Although Moses saw flames, the bush did not burn up, so he went over to investigate.

God called to Moses from within the bush and told him he had seen the misery of the Jews in Egypt and was concerned about their suffering. He told Moses to go to Pharaoh and tell him to let the Israelites go and then to lead God's people out of Egypt.

Moses did not want to do what God asked him to do. He felt inadequate. The job was too big. He was a murderer. Who was he to go before Pharaoh? Why would the most powerful ruler in the land listen to an insignificant sheepherder? I can't do this, he told God. I'm not a natural leader. I'm not a strong speaker. No one will listen to me. Pick someone else.

God told Moses he would be with him. He promised he would perform miracles through Moses to prove to Pharoah and the Israelites that God had sent him. He promised to help Moses speak and to give him the words to say.

But even with God's assurances, Moses still tried to get out of doing what God wanted. "Pardon your servant, Lord," he said. "Please send someone else" (Exodus 4:13).

I can relate to Moses. I have felt God calling me to do things I didn't want to do—small things like visiting a sick friend in the hospital when my selfish self never wanted to step foot inside a hospital again—and big things, like consenting to a heart transplant and writing this memoir.

I have felt unprepared, unworthy, and inadequate. I have tried to reason with God and talk him into choosing someone else. I've asked him to pick different tasks for me to perform. Each time I argued with God, I rationalized my stubborn refusal to obey with reasons he was making a mistake in picking me.

By focusing on myself and my inadequacy, I forgot the most important point. By myself, I am unprepared, unworthy, and inadequate. But God is sufficient for anything and everything. If he asks me to do something for him, he will provide the means for me to accomplish his will. Not through my strength, but through his. Like Moses, I learned that even though I wouldn't have chosen the path God chose for me, he gave me the courage, strength, and means to accomplish his will.

God sent Aaron, Moses's brother, to help him on his journey. Moses reluctantly faced his insecurity and fear, responded to God's call, and returned to Egypt. He gained courage because God promised to be with him, and Moses's bravery then inspired the Jewish slaves to follow him. Moses succeeded in God's plan for him and led the Israelites out of their bonds of slavery and into the promised land.

No matter how difficult a situation may appear, if we ask God for help—strength, peace, perseverance—he will provide all we need to accomplish his plan for us. He promises to be with us in our trials, as he was with Moses, if we trust him and call out to him in prayer.

DAVID

In you, LORD my God, I put my trust. (Psalm 25:1)

David was born in Bethlehem, the youngest of Jesse's eight sons. As a boy, David worked as a shepherd and watched over his father's sheep. He protected the flock from dangerous predators and killed any lion or bear that disturbed the flock. In this role, David grew physically strong and agile. As a youth, he also developed a talent for music and could sing, write songs, and play musical instruments.

When David was approximately ten to twelve years old, the king of Israel, King Saul, disobeyed God, and God rejected him as king. God sent the prophet Samuel to Bethlehem and told him to go to a man named Jesse, for God had chosen one of Jesse's sons to be king.

Samuel thought Jesse's oldest son, Eliab, was surely God's choice as the future king. But the Lord told Samuel he does not look at a person's outward appearance. He looks at the heart. Seven of Jesse's sons were brought before Samuel, and Samuel rejected each one. Finally, Jesse sent for his youngest son, David, who was tending the sheep.

God chose David as the next king, and Samuel anointed the boy with oil.

King Saul was experiencing spiritual oppression at this time, some sort of anxiety or mental anguish. His advisers suggested finding a musician whose music would calm the king's tormented spirit. One of the king's servants suggested David, and the king sent for him. David played the harp for Saul, and his music soothed the king. So, David entered the king's service as an armor-bearer and musician and divided his time between protecting his father's sheep and working for King Saul.

The Philistine army gathered their forces for war against the Israelites. The two armies faced off, the Philistines on one hill, the Israelites on another, with a valley between them. Goliath, a champion for the Philistines, challenged the Israelites. He told them to choose one man to fight him, and if the Israelite won, the Philistines would become their subjects. But if Goliath won, the Israelites would become subjects of the Philistines. Goliath stood over nine feet tall. He wore bronze armor and carried a javelin and a spear. When King Saul and the Israelites heard Goliath's taunts, they were terrified. No one could defeat such a beast.

For forty days, the two armies faced off and Goliath repeated his threat. Three of Jesse's sons had followed King Saul into battle and were camped with the Israelite army. Jesse told David to go to the Israelite camp, check on his brothers, and deliver food to them. David reached the Israelite camp as the soldiers were taking their battle positions. As David chatted with his brothers, Goliath stepped out from the enemy camp and shouted his daily challenge.

When David heard Goliath insulting the Israelites, he volunteered to fight the giant. But King Saul scoffed at the idea of a mere boy fighting the mighty warrior. David told the king how he watched over his father's sheep and killed wild animals when they threatened the flock. Then David said, "The LORD who rescued me from the paw of the lion and the paw of the bear will rescue me from the hand of this Philistine" (1 Samuel 17:37). Saul reluctantly agreed and sent David out to face Goliath.

David chose five smooth stones from the stream and placed them in the pouch of his shepherd's bag. Then he grabbed his sling and walked out to face his adversary. David and Goliath ran toward each other. David took a stone out of his shepherd's bag, loaded his sling, and fired. The stone struck Goliath on the forehead, and he fell to the ground and died.

David was an unlikely hero to save the Israelites from the Philistine army—he was a mere boy. But God chose him and used him for his glory because of his faith. David knew he would defeat Goliath because he knew God was with him. David's faith became the defining characteristic of his life.

After David killed Goliath, his popularity spread throughout Israel. King Saul became jealous of David and plotted to have him killed. David spent many years fleeing from Saul, but in spite of the hardships he encountered, he never lost his faith in God. David looked for God's purpose in his suffering and prayed for the courage to live a righteous life. He knew God was good. He knew God loved him. And he knew God's plan for him was perfect, even when life was a struggle.

Many years later, David became king of Israel. He reigned for forty years, and although he was Israel's greatest king, he was far from perfect. David noticed a beautiful woman named Bathsheba and slept with her even though they were both married to other people. Bathsheba became pregnant, and David tried to hide his adultery by sending her husband Uriah to the war's front lines where fighting was fierce, hoping he would be killed in battle. Uriah died in combat, David married Bathsheba, and she gave birth to a son who died in infancy.

David recognized his sin with Bathsheba and was filled with remorse. He cried bitterly and asked God to forgive him. Despite his flaws, David loved God and was loved by him. God knew David was not perfect—he was human, a sinner like you and me. But David sincerely asked for forgiveness when he sinned, and God always forgave him.

David wrote many of the Psalms of the Bible, and the feelings he expressed in his psalms are just as applicable today as they were when he wrote them. His words comfort me when I am faced with challenges, when I make mistakes, and when I cry out to God and don't hear an answer. David reminds me to trust God through all the ups and downs of life. He reminds me that God's love is eternal. Even when I turn my back on him and sin, God is faithful.

He will never turn his back on me.

JESUS

Come to me, all you who are weary and burdened, and I will give you rest. (Matthew 11:28)

Jesus Christ, the son of God, is the ultimate example of perseverance. His story is told in the four Gospels of the Bible: Matthew, Mark, Luke, and John.

Jesus lived a perfect life, a sinless life, and yet he knew pain. He was rejected by those he came to save. His closest friends deserted him in his darkest hour. He faced humiliation, torture, and an excruciating death. And he did it voluntarily. For us.

Jesus was fully God and fully human. As God, he knew what was going to happen to him. He knew he would endure unimaginable pain and carry the sins of the world to his death. Like any rational person, Jesus did not want to suffer. But he did. For us.

The night before his crucifixion, Jesus prayed and asked God to take away his suffering. "*Abba*, Father," he said, "everything is possible for you. Take this cup from me" (Mark 14:36). As he prayed, Jesus was in physical and emotional anguish. The Bible describes how his sweat was like drops of blood falling to the ground. He could have walked away from the greatest pain a human being has ever endured, gone back to heaven, and let the human race destroy itself with no hope of redemption.

But he didn't. He continued to pray to his father in heaven and submitted to God's plan. "Yet not as I will, but as you will" (Matthew 26:39). God did not take away his son's pain. Jesus suffered horribly on the cross. But he trusted his heavenly father and submitted to his plan in love. He stayed, suffered, and died. For us.

Jesus was betrayed by Peter, one of his closest friends. He was nailed to a cross, mocked by a crowd, and abandoned by the people he loved. He felt alone and completely vulnerable. On the cross, he again cried out to his father, "My God, my God, why have you forsaken me" (Matthew 27:46)? When Jesus died on the cross, all our sins were placed on him. In that moment, as he carried the sins of the world, Jesus was separated from his father. In the agony of that moment, he cried out in pain. Yet he endured it. For us.

Jesus knows suffering, and he won't abandon us in ours. He is the greatest example of perseverance the world has ever seen. The Bible tells us that while Jesus was on earth, he was tempted in every way a person can be tempted, and he suffered in every way a person can suffer. But he knew his suffering was temporary, and he knew it was part of God's plan. Jesus persevered because he knew God's plan was perfect. He knew God loved him. And he knew God loves us and wants to spend eternity with us in heaven. Jesus was willing to die an excruciating death to guarantee eternal life for us.

Jesus persevered through every conceivable adversity a person can face, and we can persevere too.

Not in our own strength, but in his.

PART III

A HISTORY OF HEART TRANSPLANTATION

Heal me, LORD, and I will be healed; save me and I will be saved, for you are the one I praise. (Jeremiah 17:14)

Heart disease is the leading cause of death for men and women worldwide. The development of cardiac drugs—cholesterol-lowering drugs, beta blockers, and blood thinners—have improved the quality of life for countless cardiac patients. During World War II, military surgeons removed shrapnel from scores of wounded soldiers' hearts. As a result of their groundbreaking work, heart surgery became a viable treatment option for certain types of heart disease. For patients with end-stage heart failure, where drugs were no longer effective and traditional surgeries were not a viable option, physicians around the world explored heart transplantation as a treatment option.

In the 1960s, Dr. Norman Shumway, a surgeon at Stanford University in California, researched transplantation by performing heart transplants on dogs. He spent eight years perfecting the procedure and saw longer and longer survival rates in the animals. By late 1967, Dr. Shumway felt confident enough in the surgery to perform a human heart transplant. He awaited a suitable donor for the heart patients in his care.

Dr. Christiaan Barnard, a cardiac surgeon in Cape Town, South Africa, had trained with Dr. Shumway in California. Dr. Barnard performed the first human heart transplant on December 3, 1967, at a hospital in Cape Town. A month later, Dr. Shumway performed America's first heart transplant on January 8, 1968. Based on their success and the media coverage surrounding the surgeries, surgeons around the world performed more than one hundred heart transplants in 1968.

Unfortunately, the two-year survival rate after transplantation was a mere 11 percent. This dismal statistic prompted medical centers around the world to abandon their transplant programs. Dr. Barnard, Dr. Shumway, and a handful of other surgeons refused to give up. They believed heart transplantation was a much-needed option for patients with end-stage heart failure and continued their transplant programs despite fierce opposition. Dr. Shumway described his work as "radical perseverance."

Dr. Shumway and his fellow transplant pioneers developed new surgical techniques for heart transplants. They refined the selection process between donors and recipients. They increased awareness of transplant surgery and as a result, increased the donor pool. They improved organ preservation techniques and heart biopsies. They learned how to identify rejection episodes and arrest them. Scientists worked alongside surgeons to create drugs to prevent rejection. They did this by developing drugs that suppress the immune system so the body of the recipient does not fight the transplanted heart as a foreign object.

In the early days of heart transplantation, individual hospitals managed all aspects of organ recovery and transplantation. If an organ could not be used at a donor hospital, there was no system in place to find matching transplant candidates in other hospitals. As a result, many lifesaving organs could not be used.

In 1984 the US Congress passed the National Organ Transplant Act. The act established a national registry to coordinate organ matching, operated by a private nonprofit agency under federal control. The United Network for Organ Sharing (UNOS) registers patients waiting for transplants and matches donated organs to those patients. The goal of the centralized UNOS system is to ensure the best possible use of donated organs to save the most lives.

When a transplant hospital accepts a person as a transplant candidate, it enters medical information such as the person's blood type, medical urgency, body size, and the location of the transplant hospital into UNOS's computerized network. When an organ procurement hospital obtains consent for an organ donation, the donor's information is also entered into the UNOS network.

Heart transplants must be performed within four to six hours after the procurement of the organ. After a family member agrees to donate a loved one's organs, the UNOS matching system goes to work. When matching donors to recipients, UNOS filters transplant candidates based on medical data and eliminates candidates who are incompatible with the donor based on blood type and other medical factors. The system then considers the distance between donor and transplant hospitals. Local candidates get organ offers before those listed at more distant hospitals. Proper organ size is also critical to a successful transplant, as the donor's heart must fit comfortably inside the recipient's rib cage. Only medical and logistical factors are used in organ matching. Personal or social characteristics such as celebrity status, income, or insurance coverage play no role in transplant priority.

Using a combination of donor and candidate information, the UNOS computer system generates a "match run," a rank-order list of candidates to be offered each organ. This match is unique to each donor and each organ. The candidates who appear highest in the ranking are those who are in most urgent need of a transplant, and/or those most likely to have the best chance of survival if transplanted.

The UNOS Organ Center places donated organs for transplantation 24 hours a day, 365 days a year.

By 1991 Dr. Shumway and his team at Stanford University had performed 687 heart transplants. More than 80 percent of his patients survived more than five years, and the longest survivor lived twenty years. Because of his perseverance, heart transplantation is now a standard medical treatment for end-stage heart failure in hospitals around the world.

Today, surgeons in the United States transplant more than 3,800 hearts each year. Only the limited availability of donor hearts restricts the number of surgeries performed. Survival rates have increased dramatically as improvements in immunosuppressive drugs have decreased rejection episodes in transplanted hearts.

Researchers continue to work on new innovations with the hope that one day, every patient who needs a heart transplant will be able to receive one. One of those innovations is called Heart-in-a-Box. Currently, donated hearts are placed on ice in a cooler after extraction and can only remain viable for four to six hours. To increase the amount of time a heart can exist outside the body, scientists have developed Heart-in-a-Box, a device that enables a heart to live outside of the body for up to twelve hours. Formally known as the Organ Care System, this device is being used and studied in major academic and medical institutions around the world.

With Heart-in-a-Box, the donated heart is connected to a portable device that mimics how it would pump within the human body. The sterile box is heated and allows the donated heart to stay warm and keep pumping until it is placed in the recipient's body. Heart-in-a-Box allows hospitals to use donated hearts from a larger geographic radius for possible transplantation. Doctors estimate using Heart-in-a-Box could significantly increase the number of available donor hearts.

Because of the shortage of donor hearts, scientists are also working to create artificial hearts. A total artificial heart (TAH) is a mechanical pump being used in some hospitals as a temporary solution for patients waiting for a heart transplant. Often called a "bridge to transplant," the polyurethane pump is placed in the chest and replaces both the left and right ventricles of the heart. A machine called a driver controls the pump from outside the body. The pump and driver work together to pump blood to and from the heart, replacing the role of a healthy heart. A TAH can help a heart patient grow strong and healthy enough to survive a heart transplant.

Scientists around the world are also researching the feasibility of transplanting animal hearts in humans. On January 11, 2022, doctors from the University of Maryland implanted a genetically modified pig heart in a 57-year-old man. Years of complicated research in xenotransplantation, transplanting animal organs into humans, led to the surgery on a man with end-stage heart disease and no other options. To reduce the risk of rejection, doctors made ten genetic modifications in the pig before removing its heart.

They blocked four genes that raised the risk of rejection and inserted six human genes responsible for immune acceptance into the pig's genome. The man lived two months with the pig heart. The US Food and Drug Administration has not yet approved xenotransplantation, but clinical trials have begun on the transplantation of pig kidneys into humans. More research is needed before clinical trials can begin on animal to human heart transplants.

The number of patients on the national heart transplant waiting list continues to climb. By checking a box on your driver's license to indicate your willingness to donate your organs, you can help ensure every patient who needs a lifesaving heart will be able to receive one.

ABOUT THE AUTHOR

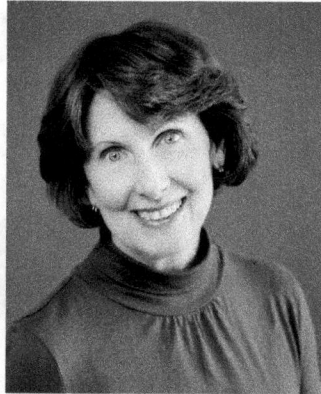

Laura B. Edge loves to read, travel, dance, and watch football games. She received her bachelor's degree in education from the University of Texas at Austin and studied abroad with the American Institute For Foreign Study in London, Paris, Rome, and Athens. Laura has taught reading and writing in middle schools and at a community college near her home in Kingwood, Texas.

She is the author of sixteen books for children and young adults and is currently working on a middle grade novel.

Learn more about Laura at www.lauraedge.com.

www.ingramcontent.com/pod-product-compliance
Lightning Source LLC
Chambersburg PA
CBHW072138270326
41931CB00010B/1804